# OCULAR NUTRITION HANDBOOK

FOR THE PRACTICING OPTOMETRIST

**Other Titles by Jeffrey Anshel, OD**

*Smart Medicine for Your Eyes*, Second Edition

*What You Must Know About*
*Age-Related Macular Degeneration*

*What You Must Know About Dry Eye*

*What You Must Know About Food and Supplements*
*for Optimal Vision Care*

*What You Must Know About Eyestrain*

# OCULAR NUTRITION HANDBOOK

## FOR THE PRACTICING OPTOMETRIST

JEFFREY ANSHEL, OD

SQUAREONE PUBLISHERS

The information and advice contained in this book are based upon the research and the personal and professional experiences of the author. They are not intended as a substitute for consulting with a healthcare professional. The publisher and author are not responsible for any adverse effects or consequences resulting from the use of any of the suggestions, preparations, or procedures discussed in this book. All matters pertaining to your physical health should be supervised by a healthcare professional. It is a sign of wisdom, not cowardice, to seek a second or third opinion.

SQUAREONE PUBLISHERS

An imprint of The Globe Pequot Publishing Group, Inc.
64 South Main Street
Essex, CT 06426
www.GlobePequot.com

Library of Congress Cataloging-in-Publication Data

ISBN 978-0-7570-0545-9 (paperback)
ISBN 978-0-7570-5545-4 (ebook)

# Contents

**CONTENTS**

*This book is dedicated to my son Casey,*
*who has always been a great inspiration to me*
*and has become a great father*
*to my beautiful granddaughter, Che.*

# Acknowledgments

NO COMPREHENSIVE TEXT CAN BE EFFECTIVELY WRITTEN BY JUST ONE person. Over the course of writing this book, as well as the years of study on ocular nutrition, I have had the honor of working with some very intelligent, dedicated and fascinating people.

A special thanks starts with an acknowledgement of my mentor, Ellen Troyer, MT, MA. Ellen was instrumental in teaching me the basics, as well as the intricacies, of ocular nutrition. Her forward thinking and willingness to share her knowledge allowed me to build a solid background for the benefit of our optometric patients, as well as the doctors who treat them.

I had the honor of knowing and working with Brian Banks of Natural Ophthalmics who was well-versed in homeopathy and shared his knowledge and support to me and the Ocular Wellness and Nutrition Society (OWNS).

Dr. A. Paul Chous is a national speaker and expert in diabetes who has also been very generous in his support of my work and as a former board member of OWNS. His contributions to the information on diabetes are greatly appreciated.

And Dr. Glen Swartwout, who is one of the original holistic optometrists in the county and is dedicated to the natural approach to ocular health.

A special recognition goes to Dr. Stuart Richer, OD, PhD who was a good friend and ardent supporter of my mission to educate doctors in the area of ocular nutrition. Stuart always challenged me to exceed my limitations and think outside the box. His belief in the need for this book was invaluable and he continues to inspire me.

I would also like to thank the members and leadership of the Ocular Wellness and Nutrition Society who are hungry for knowledge concerning nutritional approaches to vision health.

This book represents the combined efforts of a number of helpful experts who commitment and knowledge were required for its message to be expressed effectively. I thank them all again for their dedication.

Of course, I would like to thank my friends and family members who continue to support my personal and professional goals.

# Preface

In 1978, I opened a practice of optometry at the "Holistic Healing Arts" clinic in Solana Beach, California. The idea of holistic (or "wholistic") healing was a *New Age* concept that included considering the body, mind and spirit in the healing process. This clinic housed a whole array of practitioners, including acupuncturists, chiropractors, nutritionists, physical therapists, masseuses, homeopaths and colon therapists just to name a few. Each one of these practitioners included nutrition as a part of their protocol. No one had ever heard of a "holistic" optometrist before. And the only thing I ever heard regarding "ocular nutrition" was that *carrots were good for your eyes.*

My idea of holistic optometry was grounded in the fact that I was offering vision therapy, which not only included helping kids with reading and learning problems, but soon involved basic vision improvement, which we now call "myopia control". I learned about the Bates Method, Syntonic therapy, Acupressure, Homeopathy and a whole new concept of visual improvement techniques. It was a great learning and growing experience. However, I had to learn about ocular nutrition myself since there were no optometric courses offering nutrition education and the whole area seemed foreign to the profession. So, if something was good to improve blood flow to an organ, it was obviously needed in the eye. If something was helpful for nerve impulse transmission, it must have been good for the eye. If something supported muscle strength or coordination, it was obviously important for the eye. And so forth…

With that influence, I learned some of the basics about nutrition and applied them to my own life. I essentially became a vegetarian, which lasted for about 20 years. I didn't do any formal studies in nutrition but just studied on my own and listened and learned from my friends, colleagues and peers. I listened to my body to see what made me feel good and what made me feel poorly. I was my own scientific experiment.

And then came the results of the National Eye Institute study called AREDS in 2001. This was the first randomized, placebo-controlled, double-blind study of the effects of nutrition on an eye disease (AMD) and it showed a positive effect. No, it didn't "cure" AMD, nor did it reverse it but it did show that it slowed the progression. The industry was all a-buzz with this new information and then the speakers at conferences started talking about how wonderful this formula was and why we should be recommending it. But, given my knowledge at the time, I felt that there had to be more to support eye health than just five ingredients.

A few years later, I realized that there was quite a bit of "stretching" of the truth about the role of nutrition in eyecare and much of it was targeted to product sales from vitamin manufacturers. I felt that the industry needed an independent research-based source for true science around ocular nutrition. I consulted with a few colleagues and supporters and we formed the Ocular Nutrition Society in early 2008. It has since expanded to be known as the Ocular Wellness and Nutrition Society (OWNS).

During this whole time (actually since optometry school), I was working on a book that was eventually published as, "Healthy Eyes, Better Vision". It was a consumer-oriented book to inform patients about all the aspects about eye care and eye health, including some basic nutrition, vision development, aging issues, vision therapy, computer viewing issues and more. The book was published in 1990 by The Body Press. However, sales of the book were dismal.

Through a patient of mine, I learned of another publisher who had "alternative health" books and contacted them with my book. They reviewed it and responded with "we know why it didn't sell". That sounded disheartening but they also came up with another concept to make a better book. Thus, I then started working on "Smart Medicine for Your Eyes", which was published in 1999 by Avery Publishing. As my luck would have it, the book hit the market at the same time that the company sold out to a larger publisher and the title was simply stuck in the back of a catalog with no media press to promote it. However, one of the partners at Avery started a new company called Square One Publishing. They gave me the opportunity to update my book and it was released in 2011. A second edition of this title was released in 2023.

The book was promoted to the general public but I soon realized that eyecare professionals were also interested in it. Since the book was not written for the eyecare professional, I then decided to revise the book into a handbook form and re-publish it as the Ocular Nutrition Handbook. My publisher suggested that it should be written for "interested professionals". That included chiropractors, functional medical doctors, physical therapists, and more. However, this latest version is written specifically for optometrists. This is something that all eye doctors can use as a reference for a variety of different eye disorders and make positive recommendations to their patients who need nutritional support for their eye health.

This book won't get "worn out" because it's an e-book. It is designed to be a chairside companion that will assist in promoting the proper nutrition to help your patients stay healthy or heal quickly if they don't. This concept is called *Integrative Optometry* whereby nutrition and lifestyle recommendations work in conjunction with medical treatments where appropriate. I truly believe that this is the future of primary eyecare.

PART I

# NUTRITION BASICS

# Introduction

BECAUSE THE EYES AND VISUAL SYSTEM ARE SUCH AN INTEGRAL PART OF the body, it makes sense that they require proper nutrition to maintain their optimal function. You might be surprised to find out that the brain and visual system, while composing only about 2 percent of your body weight, use up about 25 percent of our nutritional intake. Let's review what nutritional support the eyes—and the body—need for optimal performance.

This chapter is designed to give you an overview of nutrition, explaining how digestion works and how it generally affects the body. While much of this is something that the eyecare professional has already learned in general physiology courses, it is reproduced here as a handy reference and background for building a working knowledge of nutrition as it applies to the visual system. In doing so, we'll discuss the macronutrients (water, carbohydrates, protein, and fats) and some selected micronutrients (vitamins and minerals) that are especially important for the practicing optometrist.

# DIGESTION, ABSORPTION, AND METABOLISM

NUTRITION INCLUDES THE PROCESS BY WHICH THE BODY DIGESTS FOOD to obtain the nutrients it needs for growth and repair purposes. Proper nutrition involves consuming foods and supplements that supply the correct nutrients in adequate amounts for optimal health. In this section, we will examine how the body processes these nutrients.

The foods eaten by humans are chemically complex and must be broken down by the body into simpler chemical forms so that they can be taken in through the intestinal walls and transported by the blood to the cells. In the cells, they provide energy and building materials to maintain human life. The processes that work together to complete these jobs are digestion, absorption, and metabolism.

## DIGESTION

Digestion is a series of physical and chemical processes that break down food in preparation for the absorption of its nutrients from the intestinal tract into the bloodstream. These processes take place in the digestive tract, which includes the mouth, pharynx, esophagus, stomach, small intestine, and large intestine.

The active materials in the digestive juices that cause the chemical breakdown of food are enzymes. Enzymes are complex proteins that are capable of inducing chemical changes in other substances without being changed themselves. Each enzyme is capable of breaking down only a single specific substance. For example, an enzyme capable of breaking down fats cannot also break down proteins or carbohydrates.

Digestion actually begins in the mouth, where the large pieces of food are broken down into smaller pieces via chewing. The salivary glands in the mouth produce saliva that moistens the food for swallowing and contains the enzyme ptyalin, which is necessary for carbohydrate breakdown. This speaks to the importance of breaking down carbohydrates quickly and thoroughly to prepare them for the digestive activity. Active chemical digestion begins in the middle portion of the stomach, where the food is mixed with gastric juices containing hydrochloric acid, water, and enzymes that break up protein and other substances. After one to four hours, muscle action pushes the food, now in a liquid form, out of the stomach and into the small intestine.

When the liquid food enters the small intestine, the pancreas secretes digestive juices that are added to the mixture. If fats are present in the food, bile from the liver and stored in the gallbladder, is secreted. The pancreas also secretes a substance that neutralizes the digestive acids in the food, as well as additional enzymes that continue the breakdown of the proteins and carbohydrates. Finally, the undigested portions of the food enter the large intestine for eventual excretion. No digestive enzymes are secreted in the large intestine, and little occurs there aside from the absorption of water.

## ABSORPTION

Absorption is the process by which nutrients—in the form of glucose from carbohydrates, amino acids from protein, and fatty acids and glycerol from fats—are taken up by the intestines and passed into the bloodstream to function in cell metabolism. Absorption takes place primarily in the small intestine. The lining of the small intestine is covered with microvilli. These microvilli contain lymph channels called lacteals and capillaries, which are the principal channels of absorption. About 60 to 70 percent of fats and fat-soluble vitamins are absorbed by the lacteals into the lymphatic system and transported to the liver. The remaining nutrients are absorbed by the capillaries into the bloodstream and transported to the liver.

In the liver, many different enzymes help to change the nutrient molecules into new forms for specific purposes. Unlike the earlier changes, which prepared the nutrients for absorption and transport, the reactions in the liver produce the actual products needed by the cells. Some of these products are used by the liver itself, but the rest are held in storage by the liver, to be released as needed into the bloodstream. From the blood, they are picked up by the individual cells and put to work.

## METABOLISM

Metabolism is the final stage of food handling. It includes all the chemical changes that nutrients undergo from the time they are absorbed until they either become a part of the body or are excreted from the body. Metabolism is the conversion of digested nutrients into building materials for living tissues or energy to meet the body's needs.

Metabolism occurs in two general phases, anabolism and catabolism, which take place simultaneously. Anabolism involves all the chemical reactions that nutrients undergo in the construction or building up of body chemicals and tissues such as blood, enzymes, hormones, and glycogen. Catabolism involves all the reactions that break down various compounds and tissues to supply energy. Energy for the cells is derived primarily from the metabolism of glucose, which combines with oxygen in a series of chemical reactions to form carbon dioxide, water, and cellular energy. The carbon dioxide and water are waste products, carried away from the cells by the bloodstream. Energy is also derived from the metabolism of essential fatty acids and amino acids, although the major purpose of amino acid metabolism is to provide material for the growth, maintenance, and repair of tissues. The waste products of essential fatty acid and amino acid metabolism are also carried away from the cells by the bloodstream.

The process of metabolism requires that the body maintain extensive systems of enzymes to facilitate the thousands of different chemical reactions that take place and to regulate the rate at which these reactions occur. These enzymes often require the presence of specific vitamins and minerals to perform their functions. For proper growth, the body needs the four basic nutrients of water, carbohydrates, protein, and fat—called macronutrients—as well as vitamins and minerals—called micronutrients. In the remainder of this chapter, we will describe these various nutrients and how they interact to supply the body and eyes with the materials they need to perform the amazing function of vision.

# THE MACRONUTRIENTS

THE MACRONUTRIENTS ARE THE ESSENTIAL INGREDIENTS AMONG THE building blocks of nutrition. They are water, carbohydrates, protein, and fat, all of which are required for the process of metabolism. Although the macronutrients are critical for life itself, there are no Federal guidelines regarding their intake, such as there are for the vitamins and minerals. All of the macronutrients are required to some degree, and are available from the foods we eat. Let's review the macronutrients, and see how they interact with our bodies to supply the fuel for life.

## WATER

Water is an essential nutrient, involved in every function of the body. It helps to transport other nutrients and waste products in and out of the cells. It is necessary for all of the digestive, absorptive, circulatory, and excretory functions of the body, as well as for the body's utilization of the water-soluble vitamins. It is also needed for the maintenance of proper body temperature. The human body is two-thirds water.

Replenishing your body's supply of water, which is continually drained through sweating and elimination, is very important. To keep your body functioning properly, it has been widely circulated that you need to drink at least eight 8-ounce glasses of quality water each day. To my knowledge, there are no actual studies that confirm that 64 ounces of water a day is a required amount but adequate hydration is always a good idea. While the body can survive without food for about five weeks, it cannot survive without water for more than five days.

## CARBOHYDRATES

Carbohydrates supply the body with the energy it needs to function. They are found almost exclusively in plant foods, such as fruits, vegetables, and legumes. Milk and milk products are the only animal foods that contain a significant amount of carbohydrates.

Carbohydrates are divided into two groups—simple and complex. The simple carbohydrates, sometimes called simple sugars, include fructose (fruit sugar), sucrose (table sugar), and lactose (milk sugar). Fruits are among the richest natural sources of simple carbohydrates. Complex carbohydrates are also made of sugars, but the sugar molecules are strung together into longer, more complex chains. The complex carbohydrates include fiber and starches. Foods rich in complex carbohydrates are vegetables, whole grains, and legumes.

Carbohydrates are the main source of blood glucose, which is a major fuel for all of the body's cells and an important source of energy for the brain and red blood cells. Except for fiber, which cannot be digested, both simple and complex carbohydrates are converted into glucose. The glucose is then either used directly to provide energy for the body or stored in the liver for future use. When a person consumes more calories than the body needs, a portion of the carbohydrates consumed may also be stored in the body as fat. Thus, when too many carbohydrates are consumed or not processed properly, excess fatty tissue accumulates and stresses the body. We'll discuss this process in more detail in the section on A Healthy Diet for Diabetes in the last chapter.

## PROTEIN

Protein is essential for growth and development. It provides the body with energy, and is needed for the manufacture of hormones, antibodies, enzymes, and tissues. It also helps to maintain the proper acid-alkaline balance in the body. When protein is consumed, it is broken down in the body into amino acids, which are the building blocks of protein. Some amino acids are considered nonessential. This does not mean that they are unnecessary, but rather that they do not have to come from the diet because they are manufactured by the body from other amino acids. The remaining amino acids are considered essential, meaning that they are not synthesized by the body and must be obtained from the diet.

Because of the importance of consuming proteins that provide all of the essential amino acids, dietary proteins are divided into two groups according to the amino acids they contain. Complete proteins, which constitute the first group, contain ample amounts of all of the essential amino acids. These proteins are found in meat, fish, poultry, cheese, eggs, and milk. Incomplete proteins, which constitute the second group, contain only some of the essential amino acids. These proteins are found in foods such as grains, legumes, and leafy green vegetables.

Although it is important to consume the full range of amino acids, both essential and nonessential, it is not necessary to get them from meat, fish, poultry, and the other complete-protein foods. In fact, because of their fat content, most of those foods should be eaten in moderation. It is possible to create complete proteins by combining various incomplete-protein foods. This is called food combining. For instance, although beans and rice are both quite rich in protein, each lack one or more of the essential amino acids. However, when you combine beans and rice with each other, or when you combine either one with any of a number of other protein-rich foods, you form a complete protein that is a high-quality substitute for meat. This is a critical concept for someone who chooses a vegetarian diet. It's not wise to simply "give up" eating meat without paying attention to the food combining to attain the proper amount of protein.

## FATS AND FATTY ACIDS

Although much attention has been focused on the need to reduce the amount of fat in the diet, the body does need some fat. During infancy and childhood, fat is necessary for normal brain development. Throughout life, it provides energy and supports growth. Fat is, in fact, the most concentrated source of energy available to the body. However, after the age of two, the body requires only small amounts of fat—much less than what is provided by the average American diet.

Fats are composed of building blocks called fatty acids. There are three major categories of fatty acids—saturated, polyunsaturated, and monounsaturated. Saturated fatty acids are found primarily in animal products, including dairy items such as whole milk, cream, and cheese, and fatty meats such as beef, veal, lamb, pork, and ham. The fat marbling that you see in beef and pork is composed of saturated fat. Some vegetable products—including coconut oil, palm kernel, oil, and vegetable shortening—are also high in saturates. The liver uses saturated fats to manufacture cholesterol. Therefore, excessive dietary intake of saturated fats can significantly raise the blood-cholesterol level, especially the level of low-density, or "bad" lipoproteins (LDLs). However, we don't get "fat" (gain excess weight) by eating fats!

Polyunsaturated fatty acids are found in the greatest abundance in corn, soybean, safflower, and sunflower oils. Certain fish oils are also high in the polyunsaturates. Unlike the saturated fats, the polyunsaturates may actually lower your total blood-cholesterol level. In doing so, however, they also have a tendency, when present in large amounts, to reduce your high-density, or "good" lipoproteins (HDLs). For this reason, the guidelines state that the intake of polyunsaturated fats should not exceed 10 percent of the total caloric intake. These oils also contain large amounts of pro-inflammatory Omega-6 fatty acids. We will review more details of the role of fatty acids in several sections below.

Monounsaturated fatty acids are found mostly in vegetable and nut oils such as olive, peanut, and canola. These fats appear to reduce the LDL blood level without affecting the HDL level in any way. However, this positive impact upon LDL cholesterol is relatively modest. The guidelines recommend that the intake of monounsaturated fats be kept between 10 and 15 percent of the total caloric intake.

Although most foods contain a combination of all three types of fatty acids, one of the types is usually predominant. Thus, a fat or oil is considered saturated or high in saturates when it is composed primarily of saturated fatty acids. Saturated fats are usually solid at room temperature, however when ingested into a body at 98.6 degrees, they will liquify. A fat or oil composed mostly of polyunsaturated fatty acids is called polyunsaturated, while a fat or oil composed mostly of monounsaturated fatty acids is called monounsaturated.

We have recently begun to increase our awareness of *trans* fats. A *trans*-fat is produced when manufacturers add hydrogen to vegetable oil—a process called hydrogenation. Hydrogenation increases the shelf life and flavor stability of foods containing these fats. Partial hydrogenation is a similar process where the action of hydrogenation is halted partially through the process so that all of the fat is not converted.

*Trans* fat can be found in vegetable shortenings, some margarines, crackers, cookies, snack foods, and other foods made with or fried in partially hydrogenated oils. Unlike other fats, the majority of *trans* fat is formed when food manufacturers turn liquid oils into solid fats like shortening and hard margarine. A small amount of *trans* fat is found naturally, primarily in dairy products, some meat, and other animal-based foods. *Trans*-fat, like saturated fat and dietary cholesterol, raises the LDL cholesterol that increases your risk for coronary heart disease. Americans consume on average 4 to 5 times as much saturated fat as *trans*-fat in their diets. Although saturated fat is the main dietary culprit that raises LDL, *trans*- fat and dietary cholesterol also contribute significantly. Fortunately, the FDA banned artificial trans fats in the US effective as of 2020. However, trans fat levels of less than 0.5 grams per service can be listed as "0" grams *trans*-fat on the food label. If the ingredients of a product list "partially hydrogenated oil", then it contains trans fats!

Essential fatty acids have been shown to be effective in managing dry eyes, so this information will be repeated in the section on Dry Eye Disease.

There has been much information in the press about the Essential Fatty Acids (EFAs). However, much of it is misguided in regard to the effects on the eyes. The most widely discussed EFAs are the Omega-3 (listed as "good") and the Omega-6 (listed as "bad") essential fatty acids. Omega-6 fatty acids are the most plentiful in our "Standard American" diet (often referred to as SAD). They are in most everything we eat that contains fat, including meat, most seed oil, dairy products and eggs. Omega-3 fatty acids are available in many seed oils and most all cold-water fatty fish. A proper balance of these fatty acids is essential to good health. The daily intake recommendation of the Institute of Medicine is 4:1 - four times as many Omega-6 fatty acids as Omega-3 fatty acids. The SAD diet has been quoted as a ratio of about 25 or 30:1.

Fatty acids are stored in every cell membrane of our body. They have two primary functions. Firstly, they ensure cellular fluidity, acting as sentinel gatekeepers for every cell—allowing vital nutrients to enter the cell and forcing destructive free radical debris out of the cells. Secondly, both Omega-6 and Omega-3 fatty acids can be converted into three different types of active molecules called prostaglandins (PGEs). Without going into too much detail, prostaglandins achieve three basic processes: reduce inflammation and inhibit blood clotting (PGE1); constrict blood vessels, increase body temperature, and encourage blood clotting (PGE2); and play an important anti-inflammatory role (PGE3). All three of these prostaglandins are important for the body to maintain its health and balance.

Two nutritional fatty acids are docosahexaenoic acid (DHA) and arachidonic acid (ARA). DHA, a long-chain omega-3 fatty acid, is found in tissues throughout the body. DHA is a major structural and functional element of all membranes in the gray matter of the brain and the retina. It is also a key component of heart tissue. DHA is important for optimal brain and eye development in infants and has been shown to support brain, eye and cardiovascular health in adults. ARA, also a long-chain omega-6 fatty acid, is the principal omega-6 in the brain, and it is abundant in other cells throughout the body. ARA is equally important for proper brain development in infants and is a precursor to a group of hormone-like substances called eicosanoids. Eicosanoids are important in immunity, blood clotting and other vital functions in the body. Humans obtain ARA by eating foods such as meat, eggs and milk, whereas DHA is found in a limited selection of foods such as fatty fish and organ meats. The body can also synthesize DHA from its precursor alpha-linolenic acid (ALA) but this process is inefficient. Both fatty acids occur naturally in breast milk and support the mental and visual development of infants. The health benefits of DHA extend from prenatal development through adult life.

Another fatty acid, eicosapentaenoic acid (EPA) is the precursor of DHA. A slightly shorter chain fatty acid, it is important in promoting an anti-inflammatory reaction. We will discuss EPA and DHA in more detail when we review the nutritional approach to dry eyes. See the chart in the Dry Eye Disease section of the next chapter.

So, what is a good dietary balance of the macronutrients? Most experts agree that a good diet consists of about 2000 calories a day. A proper balance consists of about 30% (600 calories) from fat–mostly mono-unsaturated oils and only 7% of which should be saturated fat, 50-60% carbohydrates (1000-1200 calories)—mostly low-glycemic index complex carbohydrates (see the section on Diets for the glycemic index discussion) and about 10-20% (200-400 calories) from protein. These amounts could certainly vary from one individual to another but are generally considered a good starting point for a healthy diet. However, if someone is already overweight or obese, then a caloric reduction (under 2000 calories a day) is warranted. (refer to the DIETS section later in this book)

# THE MICRONUTRIENTS

Just like the macronutrients, vitamins and minerals are essential to life. While they are also considered nutrients, they are needed in such small amounts compared to the macronutrients that they are called micronutrients.

Because vitamins and minerals are so necessary for health, the U.S. Food and Nutrition Board of the National Research Council (NRC) has formulated recommended consumption levels, called the Recommended Daily Allowances (RDAs). But the amounts cited in these recommendations usually are adequate for maintaining a minimal level of health—that is, freedom from disease—rather than optimal health. Therefore, any adult not suffering from a specific disorder should obtain more than the RDAs of the vitamins and minerals from food and/or supplement sources. People who are active or exercise, are under great stress, are on restricted diets, are mentally or physically ill, take medication, are recovering from surgery, or smoke or consume alcoholic beverages all need higher than the normal amounts. Women who take oral contraceptives also need increased amounts.

## VITAMINS

Vitamins are essential to life. They contribute to good health by regulating the metabolism and assisting the biochemical processes that release energy from digested food. They are classified either as water-soluble or fat-soluble. The water-soluble vitamins must be taken into the body daily, as they cannot be stored and are excreted within one to four days (some sooner).

These include the B vitamins and vitamin C. The fat-soluble vitamins can be stored for longer periods of time in the body, in fatty tissues and the liver. These include vitamins A, D, E, and K. The body needs both the water-soluble and fat-soluble vitamins for proper functioning.

## VITAMIN A

Of all the micronutrients that are important to visual function, vitamin A is probably the most well-known. Vitamin A is a fat-soluble vitamin that occurs in nature in a variety of chemical forms. It is found as retinol in animal tissues. It is found as beta-carotene in plants, with the highest amounts present in fruits such as apricots and cantaloupes, and in vegetables such as carrots, pumpkins, sweet potatoes, spinach, squash, and broccoli. While retinol is readily absorbed as-is by the body, beta-carotene must be broken down before it can function as a vitamin. See "beta-carotene" in the section on carotenoids.

Vitamin A is the molecule in the retina that is responsible for the transformation of light energy into nerve impulses. It is therefore critical in the function of the eye. A lack of vitamin A can cause some forms of nyctalopia. Since vitamin A is also necessary for the maintenance of the mucous lining of epithelial cells in various tissues including the eye, it is important for the support of a proper tear level and prevention of dry eye disease.

Vitamin A additionally enhances immunity, may heal gastrointestinal ulcers, protects against pollution and cancer formation, and assists in the maintenance and repair of mucous tissue. It is important in the formation of bones and teeth, aids in fat storage, and protects against colds, influenza, and infections of the kidneys, bladder, lungs, and mucous membranes. Vitamin A also acts as an antioxidant.

The upper intestinal tract is the primary area of absorption of vitamin A, since it is here that fat-splitting enzymes and bile salts convert carotene into a usable nutrient. This conversion is stimulated by thyroxine, an amino acid obtained from the thyroid gland.

Approximately 90 percent of the body's vitamin A is stored in the liver, with small amounts deposited in the fat tissues, lungs, kidneys, and retinas of the eyes. Under stressful conditions, the body uses this reserve supply if it doesn't receive enough vitamin A from the diet. Gastrointestinal and liver disorders, infections of any kind, or any condition in which the bile duct is obstructed can limit the body's capacity to retain and use vitamin A. Factors affecting the absorption of vitamin A include the amount of the nutrient consumed, the influence of other substances present in the intestines, and the amount of the vitamin stored in the body. For these reasons, the recommended dietary amounts vary for each individual.

The most common clinical sign of vitamin A deficiency is xerophthalmia, which develops after plasma retinol has been low and the eye's vitamin A reserves have become depleted. The first sign is nyctalopia, or night blindness, as a result of low rhodopsin levels in the retina. Vitamin A deficiency is one of the top causes of preventable blindness in children, especially in third world countries. A deficiency of vitamin A may be apparent if there is dry eyes, hair or skin, is present Poor growth is another symptom. Other possible results of a vitamin A deficiency are abscesses in the ears; insomnia; fatigue; reproductive difficulties; sinusitis; pneumonia, frequent colds, and other respiratory infections; skin disorders including acne; and weight loss.

The issue of vitamin A is a controversial topic in the eyecare industry. Taking large amounts of vitamin A over long periods of time can be toxic to the body, mainly the liver. The RDAs for vitamin A are 1,500 international units (IU) for infants and children up to four years old, 3,000 IU for children from four to twelve years old, and 5,000 IU for children over twelve years old and adults. These suggested amounts increase during disease, trauma, pregnancy, and lactation. The requirements vary for people who smoke, who live in highly polluted areas, who easily absorb vitamin A, and who have pneumonia or nephritis (kidney inflammation). Increased intakes of vitamins C and E will help to prevent excessive oxidation of stored vitamin A.

Research indicates that no more than 50,000 IU per day of vitamin A can be utilized by the body except in therapeutic cases, where up to 100,000 IU is recommended. It has been suggested that the best level is somewhere between 25,000 and 50,000 IU per day. However, do not take an excess of vitamin A without first consulting a patient's physician. Toxic levels of vitamin A are associated with abdominal pain, amenorrhea, enlargement of the liver and/or spleen, gastrointestinal disturbances, hair loss, itching, joint pain, nausea and vomiting, water on the brain, and small cracks and scales on the lips. Vitamin C can help prevent the harmful effects of vitamin A toxicity. Overdose is unlikely with beta-carotene, although if one takes too much, their skin may turn slightly yellow-orange in color. It is important to take only natural beta-carotene or a natural carotenoid complex. This rarely happens with over-ingestion of carrots but can be a side effect of taking a vitamin supplement with beta-carotene being listed as the source of vitamin A.

Unfortunately, many misinformed people associate vitamin A retinol with the outdated ATBC and CARET studies and now refuse to take or recommend multiples that contain efficacious amounts of either pre-formed retinol, or pro-formed beta-carotene. This decision can quickly lead to a dramatic decrease in night vision and a host of wound healing and other immune system maladies in vitamin A deficient older people.

In spite of the more recently published science, a few ophthalmic vitamin manufacturers continue to bring "smokers" macular degeneration formulations to market, which include no, or miniscule, amounts of vitamin A retinol, and no beta-carotene. Some of these companies even go so far as to suggest that the substitution of lutein for beta-carotene to be appropriate. This can be compared to substituting apples for oranges. Lutein is, in fact, a very important player in the outer edges of the macula pigment and should be included in eye specific multiples for that reason. The xanthophyll carotenoids (lutein and zeaxanthin) have virtually no ability to convert to vitamin A, nor do they perform the same antioxidant functions as the hydrocarbon carotenoid, beta-carotene. Therefore, to suggest that the inclusion of lutein in a multiple is a good substitution for a vitamin as important to the eye and body as Vitamin A is not scientifically sound. However, the bottom line for eye health in general is to get your patients to *stop smoking*!

Vitamin A has been successfully used in treating several eye disorders, including Bitot's spots, blurred vision, true night blindness, and cataracts. Therapeutic dosages of vitamin A are necessary for the treatment of cataracts, dry eye syndrome and some forms of conjunctivitis.

## VITAMIN-B COMPLEX

All the B vitamins are water-soluble substances that can be cultivated from bacteria, yeasts, fungi, or molds. The known B-complex vitamins are B1 (thiamine), B2 (riboflavin), B3 (niacin), B5 (pantothenic acid), B6 (pyridoxine), B12 (cyanocobalamin), biotin, choline, folic acid, inositol, and para-aminobenzoic acid (PABA). The grouping of these water-soluble compounds under the term "B-complex" is based upon their common sources, their close relationship in vegetable and animal tissues, and their functional relationships.

The B-complex vitamins are active in providing the body with energy, basically by converting carbohydrates into glucose, which the body burns to produce energy. They are vital in the metabolism of fats and protein. In addition, the B vitamins are necessary for the normal functioning of the nervous system, and may be the single most important factor in the health of the nerves. They are essential for the maintenance of muscle tone in the gastrointestinal tract, and for the health of the skin, hair, eyes, mouth, and liver.

All of the B vitamins are natural constituents of brewer's yeast, liver, and whole-grain cereals. Brewer's yeast is the richest natural source of the B-complex group. Another important source of the B vitamins is intestinal bacteria. These bacteria grow best on milk sugar and small amounts of fat in the diet.

Because of the water-solubility of the B-complex vitamins, any excess vitamin is excreted rather than stored. Therefore, the B vitamins must be continually replaced. All of the B vitamins, when mixed with saliva, are readily absorbed. Sulfa drugs, barbiturates, insecticides, and estrogen can create a condition in the digestive tract that can destroy the B vitamins. Certain B vitamins are lost through perspiration.

The most important thing to remember is that all of the B vitamins should be taken together. They are so interrelated in function that a large dose of any one of them may be therapeutically valueless or may cause a deficiency of other B vitamins. In nature, we find the B-complex vitamins in yeast and green vegetables, but nowhere do we find a single B vitamin isolated from the rest. The need for the B-complex vitamins increases during infection and stress. Alcoholics and individuals who consume excessive amounts of carbohydrates require higher intakes of the B vitamins for proper metabolism. Coffee uses up the B vitamins. Children and pregnant women need extra B vitamins for normal growth.

The B vitamins are so meagerly supplied in the Standard American diet that it might be that every person in this country lacks some of them. If your patients are tired, irritable, nervous, depressed, or even suicidal, suspect a vitamin B deficiency. Gray hair (prematurely), baldness, acne and other skin problems, poor appetite, insomnia, neuritis, anemia, constipation, and a high cholesterol level also are indicators of a vitamin B deficiency. One reason there is such a great vitamin B deficiency in the American population is that we eat so much processed food from which the B vitamins have been removed. Another reason for the widespread deficiency is the high amount of sugar we consume. Sugar and alcohol destroy the B-complex vitamins.

The B vitamins have been used in the treatment of barbiturate overdose, alcoholic psychosis, and drug-induced delirium. An adequate dose has been found to control migraine headaches and attacks of Meniere's syndrome. Some heart abnormalities have responded to the use of the B-complex because the nerves affecting the heart need the B-complex vitamins for proper functioning. Massive doses of the B-complex vitamins have been used to treat polio, to improve the condition of hypersensitive children who fail to respond favorably to medications such as Ritalin, and to improve cases of shingles. Nervous individuals and persons working under tension can greatly benefit from taking larger than normal doses of the B vitamins. They may also help beriberi (caused by a vitamin B1 deficiency), pellagra (caused by a deficiency of vitamin B3, specifically nicotinic acid), constipation, burning feet, tender gums, eyelid twitching, diplopia, fatigue, lack of appetite, skin disorders, cracks at the corners of the mouth, anemia, and dry, burning eyes.

## Vitamin B1 (Thiamine)

Vitamin B1, also known as thiamine, is a water-soluble vitamin that combines with pyruvic acid to form a coenzyme necessary for the breakdown of carbohydrates into glucose, which is then oxidized by the body to produce energy. Thiamine is vulnerable to heat, air, and water in cooking. It is a component of the germ and bran of wheat, the husk of rice, and that portion of all grains which is commercially milled away to give the grain a lighter color and finer texture.

Thiamine enhances circulation, assists in the formation of blood, and aids in the production of hydrochloric acid, which is important for proper digestion. Thiamine also optimizes cognitive activity and brain function. It has a positive effect on energy, growth, appetite, and learning capacity, and is needed for muscle tone in the intestines, stomach, and heart. It also acts as an antioxidant, protecting the body from the degenerative effects of aging, alcohol consumption, and smoking.

Thiamine deficiency can lead to optic neuritis, as well as to impairment of the central nervous system. The first signs of thiamine deficiency include easy fatigue, loss of appetite, irritability, and emotional instability. If the deficiency is not addressed, confusion and loss of memory appear, followed closely by gastric distress, abdominal pain, and constipation.

The RDA for thiamine is 1.1 to 1.4 milligrams per day. A thiamine intake of 1.4 milligrams daily is recommended during pregnancy and lactation. The need for thiamine increases during severe diarrhea, fever, stress, and surgery. Thiamine has no known toxic side effects.

The richest food sources of thiamine include brown rice, egg yolks, fish, legumes, liver, pork, poultry, rice bran, wheat germ, and whole grains.

Other sources are asparagus, brewer's yeast, broccoli, Brussels sprouts, dulse, kelp, most nuts, oatmeal, plums, dried prunes, raisins, spirulina, and watercress. Herbs that contain thiamine include alfalfa, bladderwrack, burdock, catnip, cayenne, chamomile, chickweed, eyebright, fennel, fenugreek, hops, nettle, oat straw, parsley, peppermint, raspberry, red clover, rose hips, sage, yarrow, and yellow dock.

## Vitamin B2 (Riboflavin)

Vitamin B2, also known as riboflavin, is a water-soluble vitamin that occurs naturally in the same foods containing the other B vitamins. Riboflavin is stable to heat, oxidation, and acid, but disintegrates in the presence of alkalis or light, especially UV light.

Riboflavin functions as part of a group of enzymes involved in the breakdown and utilization of carbohydrates, fats, and protein. It is necessary for cell respiration because it works with enzymes in the utilization of cell oxygen. Riboflavin supports mitochondrial energy production by stimulating metabolism of fats, carbohydrates, and proteins. It is required for red blood cell formation and respiration, antibody production, growth and reproduction. It's also solely responsible for the fluorescent-yellow color in urine of people who supplement with high dose B-complex vitamins.

It also helps in the prevention of many types of eye disorders, including conjunctival injection, itching or burning eyes, cataracts and photophobia. A riboflavin deficiency is linked to the formation of neovascularization of the cornea. Age-related cataract has proven to increase in those who are vitamin B2 deficient. One Australian study of both men and women suggested the incident of age-related cataract was 50% less likely to have cataracts in those in the highest riboflavin intake than those in the lowest riboflavin intake.

Riboflavin drops and ultraviolet light exposure are now being used in the process of corneal crosslinking (CCR) to treat patients with progressive keratoconus.

Riboflavin has also been used in a number of studies to address the impaired mitochondrial oxygen metabolism in the brain linked to chronic migraine headaches. Although the findings are preliminary, data suggests that riboflavin supplementation might be a useful therapy in migraine prevention. It is also necessary for the maintenance of good vision, skin, nails, and hair. Under-nourished women at the end of pregnancy often suffer from conditions such as visual hallucinations, burning eyes, excessive tearing, and fluctuating vision.

Ariboflavinosis is the clinical name for vitamin B2 deficiency. It is rarely found in isolation and occurs frequently in combination with deficiencies of other water-soluble vitamins. Riboflavin deficiency is the most common vitamin deficiency in the United States. Symptoms can include, sore throat, redness and swelling of the lining of the mouth and throat, cracks or sores on the outside of the lips and corners of the mouth, inflammation and redness of the tongue, and moist scaly skin particularly affecting the scrotum or labia majora and the nasolabial folds. This deficiency can result from long-established faulty dietary habits, food idiosyncrasies, alcoholism, arbitrarily selected diets used for the relief of digestive problems, and/or prolonged dietary restriction.

The RDA for riboflavin is 1.6 milligrams for adult males and 1.2 milligrams for adult females. During pregnancy and lactation, the requirement goes up to 1.5 milligrams and 1.7 milligrams, respectively. According to the Food & Nutrition Board at the Institute of Medicine, no toxic or adverse effects of high supplemental riboflavin intake in humans are known. However, excessive amounts of B2 makes the retina extremely sensitive to light and prolonged ingestion of large doses of any one of the B-complex vitamins, including riboflavin, may result in high urinary losses of the other B vitamins. Therefore, it is important to take a complete B-complex along with any single B vitamin.

Fortified cereals, milk, cheese, eggs, almonds, salmon, chicken, beef, broccoli, asparagus, spinach and fortified breads are the main dietary sources of riboflavin.

## Vitamin B3 ...in)

## Vitamin B3 (Niacin)

Niacin (nicotinic acid) is another member of the B-complex family of vitamins, and is also water-soluble. It is more stable than either thiamine or riboflavin, and is remarkably resistant to heat, light, air, acids, and alkalis. As a coenzyme, niacin assists enzymes in the breakdown and utilization of protein, fats, and carbohydrates. Niacin is effective at improving circulation and increasing the HDL cholesterol level. It is vital to the proper function of the nervous system, and for the formation and maintenance of healthy tongue and digestive system tissues, and skin.

Relatively small amounts of pure niacin are present in most foods. The niacin "equivalent" listed in dietary tables refers either to pure niacin or to tryptophan, an amino acid that can be converted into niacin by the body. Lean meats, poultry, fish, and peanuts are rich sources of both niacin and tryptophan, as are such dietary supplements as brewer's yeast, wheat germ, and desiccated liver. Niacin is difficult to obtain except from these foods.

Nicotinamide riboside (NR) is an alternative form of vitamin B3. Like other forms of vitamin B3, NR is converted by your body into nicotinamide adenine dinucleotide (NAD+), a coenzyme or helper molecule. NAD+ acts as fuel for many key biological processes, such as: converting food into energy, repairing damaged DNA, fortifying cells' defense systems, and setting your body's circadian rhythm. Unfortunately, the amount of NAD+ in your body naturally falls with age. Low NAD+ levels have been linked to health concerns like aging and chronic illnesses, such as diabetes, heart disease, Alzheimer's disease and macular degeneration.

NR supplements have quickly become popular because they appear to be especially effective at raising NAD+ levels. NR is also found in trace amounts in cows' milk, yeast and beer. The RDAs suggest that the daily allowance of niacin be based on caloric intake, with 6.6 milligrams of niacin recommended for every 1,000 calories. There have been no toxic side effects reported for niacin, but taking extremely large doses can cause tingling and itching sensations, intense flushing of the skin, and throbbing in the head. There is also a possibility of developing cystoid maculopathy. This condition is reversible when the overdose is stopped. The maximum suggested dose for treatment of cholesterol is 1000 mg/day. If used for this, have the patient start with a 500 mg dose at bedtime (with some food in the stomach) for about a month. Gradually add another 500 mg pill for another month and then re-check HDL levels. Most times, this amount will be adequate for cholesterol control. Most people will sleep through the skin flush. The "no-flush" form of niacin (niacinamide) will not work for HDL modification.

Excessive consumption of sugar and starches depletes the body's supply of niacin, as does taking certain antibiotics. The symptoms of niacin deficiency are many. In the early stages, they include muscular weakness, general fatigue, loss of appetite, indigestion, and various skin eruptions. Niacin deficiency may also cause bad breath, small ulcers, canker sores, insomnia, irritability, nausea, vomiting, recurring headaches, tender gums, strain, tension, and deep depression.

### Vitamin B5 (Pantothenic Acid)

Pantothenic acid, also known as vitamin B5 is required for the conversion of carbohydrates, fats, and protein into usable energy for the body. It is necessary for the synthesis of red blood cells, steroid metabolism, and is vital in the synthesis of fatty acids, cholesterol, and other biological compounds. It is the precursor of coenzyme A (CoA), which is necessary for mitochondrial ATP energy production.

Pantothenic acid deficiency results in diminished adrenal gland function. A variety of metabolic problems will also manifest themselves. Fatigue is common along with depression, and problems associated with the digestive system. There will also be loss of nerve function, and problems with blood sugar metabolism, with hypoglycemia being the most common. Pantothenic acid deficiency can reduce immune system responses, increasing the risk of infection. Other symptoms include skin problems, insomnia, lack of coordination, muscle cramps and worsening of allergy symptoms.

Small quantities of pantothenic acid are found in most foods. The major food source of pantothenic acid is in meats, although the concentration found in food animals' muscles is only about half that in humans' muscles. Whole grains are another good source of the vitamin, but milling often removes much of the pantothenic acid, as it is found in the outer layers of whole grains. Vegetables, such as broccoli and avocados, also have an abundance of the acid. In animal feeds, the most important sources of the vitamin are rice, wheat bran, alfalfa, peanut meal, molasses, yeasts, and condensed fish solutions. The most significant sources of pantothenic acid in nature are cold water fish ovaries and royal jelly.

The derivative of pantothenic acid, pantothenol, is a more stable form of the vitamin and is often used as a source of the vitamin in multivitamin supplements. Another common supplemental form of the vitamin is calcium pantothenate. Calcium pantothenate is often used in dietary supplements because, as a salt, it is more stable than pantothenic acid in the digestive tract, allowing for better absorption.

Possible benefits of supplementation with doses of 2 g/day of calcium pantothenate have been found to reduce the duration of morning stiffness as well as the degree of disability and pain severity in rheumatoid arthritis patients. Although the results are inconsistent, supplementation may improve oxygen utilization efficiency and reduce lactic acid accumulation in athletes.

## Vitamin B6 (Pyridoxine)

Vitamin B6 is a water-soluble vitamin consisting of three related compounds—pyridoxine, pyridoxal, and pyridoxamine. It is required for the proper absorption of vitamin B12, and for the production of hydrochloric acid and magnesium. Pyridoxine plays an important role as a coenzyme in the breakdown and utilization of carbohydrates, fats, and protein. It is required for the production of antibodies and red blood cells. In addition, it facilitates the release of glycogen for energy from the liver and muscles. Vitamin B6 is converted to pryridoxal-5 phosphate, which is directly involved in mitochondrial biosynthesis

Vitamin B6 helps to maintain the balance between sodium and potassium, which regulate the body fluids and promote the normal functioning of the nervous and musculoskeletal systems. The best sources of vitamin B6 are meats and whole grains, specifically desiccated liver and brewer's yeast.

According to the RDAs, the daily allowance of vitamin B6 is based on protein intake. Adults need 2.0 milligrams of pyridoxine for every 100 grams of protein they consume per day. Children need 0.6 to 1.2 milligrams for every 100 grams of protein they consume. The need for vitamin B6 doubles during pregnancy, lactation, exposure to radiation, cardiac failure, aging, and use of oral contraceptives.

Approximately 10% of the US population consumes less than half of the RDA for vitamin B6. Epidemiological studies have indicated an association between B6 deficiency and increased cancer. In cases of vitamin B6 deficiency, there is low blood sugar and low glucose tolerance and insulin sensitivity. Deficiency may also cause loss of hair, water retention during pregnancy, cracks around the mouth and eyes, numbness and cramps in the arms and legs, slow learning, visual disturbances, neuritis, arthritis, heart disorders, and increased urination.

### Vitamin B9 (Folate)

Folate, formerly known as folacin and sometimes vitamin B9, is the generic term for naturally occurring food folates and folates in dietary supplements and fortified foods, including folic acid. Folate is a B vitamin that occurs naturally in foods, while folic acid is the synthetic version of folate that's added to foods and supplements. The terms are often used interchangeably.

One of the most important folate-dependent reactions is the conversion of homocysteine to methionine in the synthesis of S-adenosyl-methionine (SAMe), an important methyl donor. Another folate-dependent reaction, the methylation of deoxy-uridylate to thymidylate in the formation of DNA, is required for proper cell division. An impairment of this reaction initiates a process that can lead to megaloblastic anemia, one of the hallmarks of folate deficiency.

Folate is naturally present in a wide variety of foods, including vegetables (especially dark green leafy vegetables), fruits and fruit juices, nuts, beans, peas, seafood, eggs, dairy products, meat, poultry, and grains. Spinach, liver, asparagus, and brussels sprouts are among the foods with the highest folate levels.

In January 1998, the U.S. Food and Drug Administration (FDA) began requiring manufacturers to add 140 mcg folic acid/100 g to enriched breads, cereals, flours, corn meals, pastas, rice, and other grain products to reduce the risk of neural tube defects (NTDs). Because cereals and grains are widely consumed in the United States, these products have become important contributors of folic acid to the American diet.

Folic acid is available in multivitamins and prenatal vitamins, supplements containing other B-complex vitamins, and supplements containing only folic acid. Common doses of folate range from 680 to 1,360 mcg (400 to 800 mcg folic acid) in supplements for adults and 340 to 680 mcg (200 to 400 mcg folic acid) in children's multivitamins.

At least 85% of folic acid is estimated to be bioavailable when taken with food, whereas only about 50% of folate naturally present in food is bioavailable. When consumed without food, nearly 100% of supplemental folic acid is bioavailable.

## Vitamin B12 (Cyanocobalamin)

B-complex member vitamin B12 is unique in that it is the first cobalt-containing substance found to be essential for longevity. In addition, it is the only vitamin that contains essential mineral elements. Vitamin B12 cannot be made synthetically, but must be grown, like penicillin, in bacteria or molds. One of the only foods in which B12 occurs naturally in substantial amounts is animal protein. Therefore, vegans and vegetarians frequently are low in vitamin B12. At the same time, high blood levels of folic acid, also common in vegetarians, can mask a vitamin B12 deficiency. Liver is the best source of B12 and kidney, muscle meats, fish, and dairy products are other good sources.

Vitamin B12 is necessary for the normal metabolism of nerve tissue, and is involved in protein, fat, and carbohydrate metabolism. Vitamin B12 is taken into the mitochondria and plays an important role in amino acid metabolism. The actions of B12 are closely related to those of four amino acids, vitamin B5, and vitamin C. Vitamin B12 also helps iron to function better in the body, and aids folic acid in the synthesis of choline.

A B12 deficiency has been shown to affect 10-15% of individuals over the age of 60 in the U.S. Patients with B12 deficiency exhibit megaloblastic anemia and often hyperhomocysteinemia, which has been associated with increasing the risk of dry AMD progressing to wet. The symptoms of a vitamin B12 deficiency may take five or six years to appear. Deficiency of the vitamin is usually due to a lack of the intrinsic factor, a glycoprotein necessary for the absorption of the vitamin. Deficiency begins with changes in the nervous system such as soreness and weakness in the legs and arms, diminished reflex response and sensory perception, difficulty walking and speaking, and jerking of the limbs. The condition of tobacco amblyopia has been improved with injections of vitamin B12, whether or not the patient stopped smoking. The symptoms of tobacco amblyopia are blackouts, headaches, and hyperopia. No cases of vitamin B12 toxicity have ever been reported.

Cyanocobalamin can scavenge superoxide similar to superoxide dismutase in cell free assays and in vitro and in vivo. Studies have confirmed that cyanocobalamin also has neuroprotective properties. The findings lend support to the hypothesis that vitamin B12 is an endogenous superoxide scavenger that, if depleted or deficient, results in optic neuropathy.

## Biotin

Biotin, another of the B vitamins, is used in cell growth, the production of fatty acids, metabolism of fats, and proteins. It also plays a role in the Krebs cycle. Biotin is also indicated for healthy hair and skin, healthy sweat glands, nerve tissue, and bone marrow, and assisting with muscle pain. It not only assists in various metabolic chemical conversions, but also helps with the transfer of carbon dioxide. Biotin is also helpful in maintaining a steady blood sugar level.

Although a deficiency of Biotin is very rare, it can happen and may result in dry scaly skin, fatigue, loss of appetite, nausea and vomiting, mental depression as well as tongue inflammation and high cholesterol. Biotin deficiency is suggested to deplete the amino acid glycine from the mitochondrial matrix.

The RDA dosage of Biotin for adults is 30 microgram (30 mcg) per day and pregnant and lactating women is 35 microgram (35 mcg) per day.

## Choline

Choline is considered one of the B-complex vitamins. It functions with inositol, also considered a B-complex vitamin, as a basic constituent of lecithin. It is present in the bodies of all living cells, and is widely distributed in animal and plant tissues. Lecithin is the richest source of choline, but other rich dietary sources are egg yolks, liver, brewer's yeast, and wheat germ.

Choline appears to be associated primarily with the utilization of fats and cholesterol in the body. It prevents fats from accumulating in the liver, and facilitates their movement into the cells. In the liver, choline combines with fatty acids and phosphoric acid to form lecithin. It is essential for the health of the liver and kidneys.

Choline is also essential for the health of the myelin sheaths of nerves and thus plays an important role in the transmission of the nerve impulses. Choline also helps to regulate and improve liver and gallbladder functioning, and aids in the prevention of gallstones. This might be an indication if someone exhibits signs of MS.

Humans can produce choline endogenously in the liver, mostly as phosphatidylcholine, but the amount that the body naturally synthesizes is not sufficient to meet human needs. As a result, humans must obtain some choline from the diet. The daily requirements for choline are 550 mg per day. The average American adult diet has been estimated to contain 500 to 900 milligrams of choline per day.

## VITAMIN C

Vitamin C, also known as ascorbic acid, is one of the most commonly discussed and studied vitamins. It is a water-soluble nutrient. Although fairly stable in acid solutions, it is normally the least stable of the vitamins, and is very sensitive to oxygen. Its potency can be lost through exposure to light, heat or air, all of which stimulate the activity of the oxidative enzymes.

The primary function of vitamin C is to maintain the body's collagen, a protein necessary for the formation of the sclera. One school of thought regarding the effects of vitamin C on the development of myopia is that since the vitamin fortifies the sclera, a lack of vitamin C for an extended period of time, especially during the high growth years, weakens the scleral structure, allowing the pressure inside the eye to expand the length of the eye, which leads to myopia. (see the section on The Myopia Diet)

Vitamin C plays a role in the healing of wounds and burns because it facilitates the formation of connective tissue in scars. Vitamin C also aids in the formation of red blood cells and the prevention of hemorrhaging. In addition, vitamin C fights bacterial infections and reduces the effects on the body of some allergens. While vitamin C is often used to try and prevent or treat the common cold, scientific research indicates that while it may slightly reduce the duration of cold symptoms, it does not effectively prevent people from catching a cold in the general population; meaning taking vitamin C regularly does not significantly lower the chance of getting a cold.

Vitamin C is present in most fresh fruits and vegetables. Natural vitamin C dietary supplements are prepared from rose hips, acerola cherries, green peppers, and citrus fruits.

The level of ascorbic acid in the blood reaches a maximum about two or three hours after the ingestion of a moderate quantity of the nutrient, then decreases as the vitamin is eliminated in the urine and through perspiration. Most vitamin C is out of the body in three to four hours. Therefore, doses of vitamin C should be broken up to several times a day, rather than a single morning intake.

Because vitamin C is a "stress vitamin," it is used up even more rapidly under stressful conditions. Humans, apes, and guinea pigs are the only animals that must obtain vitamin C from their food because they are unable to meet the body's needs by synthesis alone. Ascorbic acid is readily absorbed from the gastrointestinal tract into the bloodstream. Two factors that influence its absorption are the manner in which the vitamin is administered and the presence of other substances in the intestinal tract. The human body, when fully saturated, contains about 5,000 mg of vitamin C, of which 30 mg are found in the adrenal glands, 200 mg in the extracellular fluids, and the rest in varying concentrations throughout the cells of the entire body.

Vitamin C promotes bone and tooth formation while protecting the dentine and pulp of teeth. Some types of viral and bacterial infections are prevented or cured by vitamin C.

It is a fact that the aqueous humor maintains a vitamin C level approximately *twenty-six times* higher than that of the blood plasma. This is considered significant in the nutrition of the lens, which depends on the aqueous fluid for its nourishment. It only stands to reason that the level of vitamin C should be upheld or increased as we age to maintain a clear and healthy lens.

High dietary intakes of vitamin C and higher plasma ascorbate concentrations have been associated with a lower risk of cataract formation in some studies. In a 5-year prospective cohort study conducted in Japan, higher dietary vitamin C intake was associated with a reduced risk of developing cataracts in a cohort of more than 30,000 adults age 45–64 years. Results from two case-control studies indicate that vitamin C intakes greater than 300 mg/day reduce the risk of cataract formation by 70%–75%. Use of vitamin C supplements, on the other hand, was associated with a 25% higher risk of age-related cataract extraction among a cohort of 24,593 Swedish women age 49–83 years. These findings applied to study participants who took relatively high-dose vitamin C supplements (approximately 1,000 mg/day) and not to those who took multivitamins containing substantially less vitamin C (approximately 60 mg/day).

In one study, Chinese adults who took daily supplements of 120 mg vitamin C plus 30 mcg molybdenum for 5 years did not have a significantly lower cataract risk. However, adults age 65–74 years who received 180 mg vitamin C plus 30 mcg molybdenum combined with other nutrients in a multivitamin/mineral supplement had a 43% significantly lower risk of developing nuclear cataracts than those who received a placebo. In the AREDS study, older individuals who received supplements of 500 mg vitamin C, 400 IU vitamin E, and 15 mg beta-carotene for an average of 6.3 years did not have a significantly lower risk of developing cataracts or of cataract progression than those who received a placebo. The AREDS2 study, which also tested formulations containing 500 mg vitamin C, confirmed these findings. (see the section on AMD).

The RDA for vitamin C is 45 milligrams for adults. However, the now-famous Dr. Linus Pauling suggested that the optimal daily intake of vitamin C for most human adults is from 2,300 to 9,000 mg. This wide range takes into account differences in weight, activity level, metabolism, ailments, and age.

Toxicity symptoms usually do not occur with high intakes of vitamin C because the body simply discharges whatever it cannot use. However, a daily intake of 5,000 to 15,000 mg may cause side effects in some people. The toxicity symptoms of vitamin C include a slight burning sensation during urination, loose bowels, and skin rashes.

The body's ability to absorb vitamin C is reduced by smoking, stress, high fever, prolonged intake of antibiotics or cortisone, inhalation of petroleum fumes, and ingestion of aspirin or other painkillers. Baking soda destroys vitamin C, as does cooking with copper utensils. The signs of deficiency include shortness of breath, impaired digestion, poor lactation, bleeding gums, weakened tooth enamel or dentine, tendency to bruising, swollen or painful joints, nosebleeds, anemia, lowered resistance to infections, and slow healing of wounds. Severe deficiency results in scurvy.

## VITAMIN D

Vitamin D is a fat-soluble vitamin that can be acquired both from food and through exposure to sunlight. It is known as the "sunshine vitamin" because the sun's UV rays activate a form of cholesterol present in the skin, converting the substance to vitamin D. The term "supplementation" has been used in the context of cholecalciferol, ergocalciferol, calcitriol, and calcitriol- all forms of vitamin D.

### Is Vitamin D a Pre-steroid or Hormone?

Vitamin D can be obtained from diet, direct sunlight, or supplementation. The most common form is synthesized in the skin after exposure to ultraviolet B radiation. Nevertheless, the thought is that vitamin D is more of a multifunctional hormone or prohormone. This is because vitamin D contributes to many processes in the body. Calcitriol has been shown to have enhancing effects on the immune system, the cardiovascular system, the endocrine system, and other metabolic pathways. There is evidence that vitamin D has also a role in depression, pain, and cancer.

Although vitamin D is commonly called a vitamin, it is not in the sense an essential dietary vitamin due to its ability to be synthesized in adequate amounts by all mammals from sunlight. Vitamin D fits within the definition of vitamin as it is "an organic compound required as a vital nutrient in tiny amounts by an organism." An organic chemical compound (or related set of compounds) is called a vitamin when it cannot be synthesized in sufficient quantities by an organism, and must be obtained from the diet.

There are two general forms of vitamin D: D2 and D3. Vitamin D3 has been shown to be more efficacious at raising serum 25(OH)D concentrations than is vitamin D2, and thus vitamin D3 is the preferred choice for supplementation. Vitamin D aids in the absorption of calcium from the intestinal tract, and in the breakdown and assimilation of phosphorus, which is required for bone formation. In the mucous membranes, it helps to synthesize enzymes that are involved in the active transport of available calcium. Vitamin D is necessary for normal growth in children, for without it, the bones and teeth do not calcify properly.

Adults also benefit from vitamin D. It is valuable for maintaining a stable nervous system, normal heart action, and normal blood clotting because all these functions are related to the body's supply and utilization of calcium and phosphorus. Vitamin D is best utilized by the body when taken with vitamin A. Fish-liver oils (such as cod-liver oil) are the best natural sources of vitamins A and D in moderate amounts.

Most of the body's need for vitamin D can be met by sufficient exposure to sunlight and ingestion of small amounts of food. However, the sun's action on the skin can be inhibited by such factors as air pollution, clouds, window glass, and clothing. The RDA for vitamin D is set at 400 IU per day, which should meet the requirements of most healthy individuals who are not regularly exposed to UV light.

Being a fat-soluble vitamin means that vitamin D can be stored in the body. Excessive blood levels of the vitamin often create a rise in the blood levels of calcium and phosphorus, and excessive excretion of calcium in the urine. This leads to calcification of the soft tissues and of the walls of the blood vessels and kidney tubules, a condition known as hypercalcemia. The symptoms of acute overdosage are increased frequency of urination, loss of appetite, nausea, vomiting, diarrhea, muscular weakness, dizziness, weariness, and calcification of the soft tissues of the heart, blood vessels, and lungs. These symptoms disappear within a few days of discontinuation of the overdosing.

It is widely recognized that most adults are deficient in vitamin D, especially those in extreme northern and southern latitudes. A deficiency of vitamin D leads to inadequate absorption of calcium from the intestinal tract and retention of phosphorus in the kidneys. The inability of the soft bones to withstand the stress of the body's weight results in skeletal malformations. Rickets, a bone disorder in children, is a direct result of vitamin D deficiency. Adult rickets, called osteomalacia, can also occur. One study showed that a vitamin D deficiency might cause myopia. In this study, low vitamin D levels were not significantly associated with myopia in children aged 5-15 years, but significant associations were found between myopia and relatively older age. An imbalance of the vitamin with calcium is likely at the root of this disorder. Other possible ocular effects are keratoconus, conjunctivitis, cataracts, and arteriosclerosis.

## VITAMIN E

Vitamin E refers to a group of eight fat-soluble compounds that include both tocopherols and tocotrienols. The eight forms are divided into two groups; four are tocopherols and four are tocotrienols. They are identified by prefixes alpha-, beta-, gamma-, and delta-with alpha-tocopherol being the most common in the North American diet. It is an antioxidant that stops the production of reactive oxygen species formed when fat undergoes oxidation. Alpha tocopherol is also the most potent and has the greatest nutritional and biological values. The tocopherols occur in the highest concentrations in cold-pressed vegetable oils, whole raw seeds and nuts, and soybeans. Wheat germ oil is the source from which vitamin E was first obtained.

Current research direction is starting to give more prominence to the tocotrienols, the lesser known but more potent antioxidants in the vitamin E family. Less than 1 percent of PubMed papers on vitamin E relate to tocotrienols but the research is growing. Numerous recent studies have demonstrated that tocotrienols possess antioxidant, anti-cholesterolemic, anti-atherosclerotic, anti-cancer, anti-tumor, anti-hypertensive, immunomodulatory and neuroprotective properties. Some studies have suggested that tocotrienols have specialized roles in protecting neurons from damage and cholesterol reduction by inhibiting the activity of HMG-CoA reductase (similar to the actions of statins).

Oral consumption of tocotrienols is also thought to protect against stroke-associated brain damage in vivo. Until further research has been carried out on the other forms of vitamin E, conclusions relating to the other forms of vitamin E, based on trials studying only the efficacy of alpha-tocopherol, may be premature.

Vitamin E plays an essential role in the cellular respiration of the muscles, especially the cardiac and skeletal muscles. It makes it possible for these muscles and their nerves to function with less oxygen, thereby increasing their endurance and stamina. It also causes vasodilation, permitting a fuller flow of blood to the heart, as well as to the other organs.

Vitamin E is effective against the formation of elevated scar tissue on the surface of the body and within the body. In ointment form, it is used on burns to promote healing and to lessen the formation of scars. As a diuretic, vitamin E helps to lower elevated blood pressure. It protects against the damaging effects of many environmental toxins.

There are several substances that interfere with, or even cause a depletion of vitamin E in the body. For example, when iron, especially the inorganic form, and vitamin E are administered together; the absorption of both is impaired. Chlorine in drinking water, ferric chloride, rancid oil or fat, and inorganic-iron compounds destroy vitamin E in the body. Mineral oil used as a laxative depletes vitamin E. Large amounts of polyunsaturated fats or oils in the diet increase the oxidation rate of vitamin E. The more unsaturated fats or oils that are consumed, the more vitamin E is necessary.

Vitamin E has many beneficial effects. It works to treat and prevent heart diseases, such as coronary thrombosis. Vitamin E can disintegrate arterial blood clots. Angina is successfully treated with alpha tocopherol. Vitamin E is beneficial to persons with atherosclerosis if used as a therapy before irreparable damage occurs. It relieves pain in the extremities, speeds up blood flow, and reduces clotting tendencies.

Vitamin E can aid in the healing of burned tissue, skin ulcers, and abrasions. It is also helpful in counteracting premature aging of the skin. It is useful to apply vitamin E to the skin in ointment form while also taking it orally, because it affects cell formation by replacing the cells on the outer layer of the skin. Vitamin E also helps to counter the gradual decline in metabolic processes during aging.

Vitamin E therapy has been suggested as beneficial in a number of other conditions, including bursitis, gout, arthritis, headaches, strabismus, varicose veins, thrombosis, phlebitis, nephritis, and even myopia. Vitamin E (400 IU) was also included in the AREDS and AREDS2 studies.

The RDA for vitamin E is based upon metabolic body size and level of polyunsaturated fatty acids in the diet, rather than upon weight or caloric intake. The requirements increase along with any increases in the amount of polyunsaturated fatty acids consumed. The RDA is 4 to 5 IU daily for infants, 7 to 12 IU for children and adolescents; 15 IU for adult males, 12 IU for adult females, and 15 IU for pregnant or lactating females. However, many nutritionists consider these allowances exceedingly low.

The first sign of a vitamin E deficiency is the rupture of red blood cells, resulting from the cells' increased fragility. A deficiency could result in a reduction of membrane stability and shrinkage of collagen. Also, a tendency toward muscular wasting or abnormal fat deposits in the muscles, and an increased demand for oxygen can occur in a deficiency state. The essential fatty acids are altered so that blood cells break down and hemoglobin formation is impaired. In addition, the body's ability to utilize several amino acids is impaired, and the level of functioning of the pituitary and adrenal glands is reduced. Iron absorption and hemoglobin formation also are impaired. A severe deficiency can cause damage to the kidneys and liver. A prolonged deficiency of vitamin E can cause faulty absorption of fat and the fat-soluble vitamins. Poor utilization of vitamin E or an increased demand for it can cause anemia.

There has been a concern in one research study in 2005 about the over-dosage of Vitamin E (400 IU) as a supplement to the diet. This isolated finding applied only to an older group of patients (over the age of 70) with a long history of heart disease, stroke or diabetes, who were also taking a combination of medications, including ACE inhibitors, calcium channel blockers, anti-platelet agents and lipid-lowering agents during the course of the study. A significant percentage of study participants were also cigarette smokers, further clouding the issue.

The Council for Responsible Nutrition continues to support the safe upper limits of vitamin E established by the Food and Nutrition Board at the Institute of Medicine. The published safe daily upper limits are 1000

IUs of synthetic Vitamin E and 1500 IUs of natural vitamin E, however under normal circumstances; a daily supplement of 200 IU is adequate.

Researchers also estimated that over 80% of the American public does not begin to get even the minimal required amount of vitamin E from their diet. One distinguished vitamin E researcher commented, "Vitamin E deficiency could make us more prone to atherosclerosis or diseases that involve an enhanced production of oxygen radicals. Renegade radical molecules can rampage throughout cells, destroying lipids, proteins, and DNA. By disarming oxygen radicals, vitamin E may act as an insurance policy against oxidative stress."

## VITAMIN K

There are three main K vitamins: $K_1$ and $K_2$ are fat soluble and can be manufactured in the intestinal tract. Vitamin $K_3$ is produced synthetically for the treatment of patients who are unable to utilize naturally occurring vitamin K because they lack bile.

If yogurt, kefir or acidophilus milk is included in the diet, the body may be able to manufacture sufficient amounts of vitamin K. In addition, unsaturated fatty acids and a low carbohydrate diet increase the amounts of vitamin K produced by the intestinal flora.

Vitamin K is necessary for the formation of pro-thrombin, which is required in blood clotting. Vitamin K is involved in phosphorylation, where phosphate is combined with glucose and is passed through the cell membranes and converted into glycogen. It is also vital for normal liver functioning and is an important vitality and longevity factor.

Vitamin K is an essential cofactor of carboxylation, making osteocalcin bind to the bone matrix; that is, it keeps calcium in the bones. Carboxylation also activates matrix GLA, a protein that prevents calcium from accumulating in arteries. This is important since most arterial plaque is made from calcium, not cholesterol.

Vitamin K is absorbed in the upper intestinal tract with the aid of bile or bile salts and is transported to the liver where it forms pro-thrombin and several related proteins involved in blood clotting. Vitamin K is stored in very small amounts and considerable quantities are excreted after administration of therapeutic doses.

Natural sources of vitamin K include kelp, alfalfa, green plants and leafy green vegetables. Cow's milk, yogurt, egg yolks, blackstrap molasses, safflower oil, fish liver oils and other polyunsaturated oils are other good sources. The most dependable supply is the intestinal bacteria. Frozen foods, rancid fats, radiation, x-rays, aspirin and industrial air pollution all destroy vitamin K. Excessive use of antibiotics can destroy the intestinal flora. Ingestion of mineral oil will cause rapid excretion of vitamin K.

The U.S. Dietary Reference Intake (DRI) for an adequate intake of vitamin K for a 25-year-old male is 120 mcg/day. The adequate intake for adult women is 90 mcg/day, for infants is 10–20 micrograms/day, for children and adolescents 15–100 mcg/day. In 2002 it was found that to get maximum carboxylation of osteocalcin, one may have to take up to 1000 mcg of vitamin K1.

A prescription form of vitamin $K_1$ called Mephyton® (phytonadione) is available.

This vitamin is clear, yellow to amber, viscous, and nearly odorless liquid. It is insoluble in water, soluble in chloroform and slightly soluble in ethanol. Mephyton® tablets possess the same type and degree of activity as naturally-occurring vitamin K and they generally exert their effect within 6 to 10 hours.

## MINERALS

Minerals are nutrients that exist in the body and in food, in organic and inorganic combinations. Approximately seventeen minerals are essential in human nutrition. Although minerals make up only 4 or 5 percent of the human body's weight, they are vital to overall mental and physical well-being. All of the tissues and internal fluids of living things contain varying quantities of minerals. Minerals are constituents of the bones, teeth, soft tissue, muscle, blood, and nerve cells. They are important in maintaining the physiological processes, strengthening the skeletal structure, and preserving the vigor of the heart, the brain, and all of the muscle and nerve systems.

Although we will discuss a number of minerals separately in the following pages, it is important to note that the actions of all the minerals within the body are interrelated; no one mineral functions without affecting the others. Physical and emotional stress can cause a strain on the body's supply of minerals. A mineral deficiency often results in illness, which may be corrected by adding the missing mineral to the diet.

## CALCIUM

Calcium is the most abundant mineral in the body. About 99 percent of the calcium in the body is deposited in the bones and teeth, with the remainder found in the soft tissues. To function properly, calcium must be accompanied by magnesium, phosphorus, and vitamins A, C, and D. Calcium is stored in mitochondria and it participates in cellular calcium signaling. Calcium is also a required co-factor in several mitochondrial proteins, including dehydrogenates (enzymes that take up hydrogen).

Calcium is also essential for healthy blood, eases insomnia, and helps to regulate the heartbeat. An important calcium partner in cardiovascular health is magnesium. Calcium assists in the process of blood clotting and helps to prevent the accumulation of too much acid or alkali in the blood. It also plays a part in muscle growth, muscle contraction, and nerve transmission. Calcium aids in the body's utilization of iron, helps to activate several enzymes, and helps to regulate the passage of nutrients in and out of cell walls.

Calcium absorption is very inefficient, with usually only 20 to 30 percent of ingested calcium absorbed. When it needs calcium, however, the body can absorb it more effectively. Therefore, the greater the need for calcium and the smaller the dietary supply, the more efficient is the absorption. Absorption is also increased during periods of rapid growth. Calcium absorption depends upon the presence of adequate amounts of vitamin D, which works with the parathyroid hormone to regulate the amount of calcium in the blood. Phosphorus is needed in at least the same amount as calcium. Vitamins A and C are also necessary for calcium absorption. Fat consumed in moderate amounts and moving slowly through the digestive tract facilitates absorption. A high intake of protein also aids in the absorption of calcium.

Certain substances inhibit calcium absorption. When excessive amounts of fat combine with calcium, the result is an insoluble compound that cannot be absorbed. Calcium combined with oxalic acid, found in chocolate, spinach, and rhubarb, makes another insoluble compound and may form into stones in the kidney or gallbladder. Other interfering factors are lack of exercise, excessive stress, and too rapid a flow of food through the intestinal tract.

One of the first signs of a calcium deficiency is a nervous affliction called tetany, which is characterized by muscle cramps, and numbness and tingling in the arms and hands. A calcium deficiency can result in bone malformation, causing rickets in children and osteomalacia in adults. Another ailment that results from calcium deficiency is osteoporosis because calcium is withdrawn from them, as well as from other body areas, faster than it is deposited. Moderate cases of calcium deficiency may lead to cramps, joint pains, heart palpitations, eyelid twitching, slow pulse rate, tooth decay, insomnia, impaired growth, and excessive irritability of the nerves and muscles.

There is a possibility of "over-calcification" with the ingestion of excessive amounts of calcium over a long period of time. This condition can lead to kidney stones, mitral valve disease and calcification of the small and large blood vessels (which includes the eyes). In addition, most of the plaques that are attributed to excess cholesterol are usually comprised more of calcium (over 50%) than cholesterol (3%).

A German study has, according to a drug company media press release, indicated that taking calcium supplements places one at a greater risk for a heart attack! Every week there are studies showing the deadly dangers of pharmaceuticals but those rarely make the media. Could all the hundreds of previous studies proving that calcium supplementation is not only safe but also essential be wrong? Let's take a closer look.

The question remains, "Are calcium supplements safe?" It depends on what form of calcium, the co-factors and how you take it.

First of all, not all calcium supplements are the same. The majority of these products are simply ground up rock in the form of coral, dolomite, eggshell, etc. and are not only very difficult to absorb but also, due to their highly alkaline pH, potentially problematic.

The root cause is a condition called calcification of the arteries—where calcium builds up on the inside of certain spots on the artery due to free radical damage to the internal muscle wall. The most common form of calcium likely to contribute to this issue is alkaline calcium or that from cheap supplements. Calcium that has been pre-acidified through chelating with an acid is much less likely to remain circulating in the bloodstream for longer periods of time.

Absorption is the key to all nutrients, especially calcium. Essential co-factors must be present to facilitate calcium absorption to not only bone but to all areas where it is essential for life. The more of these co-factors present together with calcium the faster it will be absorbed to the tissues where it is needed.

One study concludes that perhaps taking calcium in higher one-shot doses as in a supplement is a big part of the problem over getting calcium throughout the day as in food. There may be some logic in that, which is why authorities have always stressed to space out calcium supplements throughout the day as only a limited amount of the mineral can be absorbed at one time. Hundreds of studies have shown that the industrialized diet does not provide all the nutrients we need for optimal health.

In the May 2012, Journal of Clinical Nephrology: "Calcium and Vitamin D3 supplements proven effective in reducing bone loss in elderly women with kidney disease". And in May 2012, Complementary Therapies in Clinical Practice: "Effects of polycystic ovary syndrome alleviated with vitamin D and calcium supplementation".

So, are calcium supplements safe? Yes, absolutely providing that you take a Full Spectrum supplement with the right form of acidified calcium together with all the co-factors for enhanced uptake and absorption. A good calcium supplement should contain chelated calcium and magnesium. It should also contain the absorption co-factors manganese, boron, copper, zinc and strontium for bone absorption. Lastly you should space your calcium supplements throughout the day and take them with meals. If done properly, calcium supplementation will continue to provide you with the many health benefits it always has and that have been shown by many studies over the last few decades.

## CHROMIUM

Chromium is an essential mineral found in concentrations of twenty parts of chromium to one billion parts of blood. It stimulates the activity of enzymes involved in the metabolism of glucose for energy and the synthesis of fatty acids and cholesterol. Chromium also appears to increase the effectiveness of insulin, thereby facilitating the transport of glucose into the cells. In the blood, it competes with iron in the transport of protein. Chromium may also be involved in the synthesis of protein through its binding action with RNA molecules.

The sources of chromium include clams, whole-grain cereals, and meats. Fruits and vegetables contain trace amounts. Brewer's yeast provides a dependable supply without the problems of high carbohydrate intake and high cholesterol levels. Chromium is difficult to absorb. Only about 3 percent of dietary chromium is retained in the body, and the amount of chromium stored in the body decreases with age.

A chromium deficiency may upset the function of insulin, and result in depressed growth rates and severe glucose intolerance in diabetics. It is also believed that the interaction of chromium and insulin is not limited to glucose metabolism, but also affects amino acid metabolism. Chromium may inhibit the formation of aortic plaques, and a deficiency may contribute to atherosclerosis. Chromium deficiency has also been shown to be a factor in the development of myopia.

## COPPER

Wilson's disease is a hereditary disorder in which the body retains too much copper. Copper is a trace mineral, which means it is essential for good health, but only a tiny amount is needed. When excess copper accumulates, it is stored in the eyes, brain, kidneys, and liver. Excess copper collecting in the liver causes cirrhosis of the liver, which is a serious, life-threatening condition. However, Wilson's disease is treatable.

Copper is found in different amounts in a wide variety of foods. Therefore, dietary restriction alone is usually not enough to control Wilson's disease. Still, it is helpful to avoid copper-rich foods as much as possible. Some of the foods rich in copper are liver, oysters, sesame seeds, cocoa powder, nuts, calamari and sunflower seeds.

Over-consumption of copper will lead to cramps, diarrhea, and vomiting in the short term, and can lead to depression, schizophrenia, hypertension, senility, and insomnia in the long term. The stomach needs to be acidic in order to absorb copper and thus antacids interfere with the absorption of copper, as do milk and egg proteins.

A link between copper and iron metabolism is well established. Copper deficiency increases dietary iron absorption, which is probably a compensatory mechanism to increase mitochondria iron production. Both copper and zinc are needed for an important antioxidant enzyme called superoxide dismutase (SOD) that helps to fight free radicals and reduce oxidative stress; the ratio between the two is vital for keeping this enzyme functioning optimally. Copper is included in the AREDS and AREDS2 studies to balance the inclusion of zinc in the formula.

## IRON

Iron is a large part of hemoglobin. Iron-deficient people tire easily because their bodies are starved for oxygen. Iron is also part of myoglobin, which helps muscle cells store oxygen. Without enough iron, ATP cannot be properly synthesized. As a result, some iron-deficient people become fatigued even when their hemoglobin levels are normal.

Although iron is part of the antioxidant enzyme catalase, iron is not generally considered an antioxidant, because too much iron can cause oxidative damage.

The most absorbable form of iron, called "heme" iron, is found in oysters, meat, poultry, and fish. Non-heme iron is also found in these foods, as well as in dried fruit, molasses, leafy green vegetables, wine, and most iron supplements. Acidic foods (such as tomato sauce) cooked in an iron pan can also be a source of dietary iron. Normal aging of the brain and neurodegenerative changes share certain pathological and physiological changes with the retina, including mitochondrial dysfunction, oxidative stress, and loss of iron balance, which naturally declines with age. It is becoming clear that many organs show morphologic, physiologic, and biochemical changes before hemoglobin levels change. Heme is synthesized in the mitochondria and the decline in synthesis could explain the loss of iron in aging.

Vegetarians eat less iron than non-vegetarians, and the iron they eat is somewhat less absorbable. As a result, vegetarians are more likely to have reduced iron stores. However, iron deficiency is not usually caused by a lack of iron in the diet alone; an underlying cause, such as iron loss in menstrual blood, often exists.

Pregnant women, marathon runners, people who take aspirin and those who have parasitic infections, hemorrhoids, ulcers, ulcerative colitis, Crohn's disease, gastrointestinal cancers, or other conditions that cause blood loss or malabsorption are likely to become deficient. Individuals who fit into one of these groups, even pregnant women, shouldn't automatically take iron supplements. Fatigue, the first symptom of iron deficiency, can be caused by many other things. A nutrition-oriented doctor should assess the need for iron supplements, since taking iron when it isn't needed does no good and may do some harm.

The current recommended daily allowance for iron is 18 mg. If a lab test confirms iron deficiency, iron supplementation is essential and the doctor must also determine the cause. Usually it's not serious (such as normal menstrual blood loss or blood donation). Occasionally, however, iron deficiency signals ulcers or even colon cancer. Many pre-menopausal women become marginally iron deficient unless they supplement with iron. Even so, the 18 mg of iron present in most multiple-vitamin/mineral supplements is often adequate. In post-menopausal women, iron is contraindicated in supplement form.

An increase in consumption of iron can increase the risk of cardiac disease, as well as retinal blood vessel issues. In general, most iron can be accumulated in a good diet and the use of iron supplements is most often not needed.

## MAGNESIUM

Magnesium is an essential mineral that accounts for about .05 percent of the body's total weight. Nearly 70 percent of the body's supply is located in the bones together with calcium and phosphorus, while 30 percent is found in the soft tissues and body fluids.

Magnesium is involved in many essential metabolic processes. Most of the body's magnesium is found inside the mitochondria in the cells, where it activates enzymes necessary for the metabolism of carbohydrates and amino acids. The mitochondria account for nearly one third of total cellular magnesium. Moderate magnesium deficiency is common, particularly among African-Americans and is associated with increased risk for hypertension and diabetes. By countering the stimulative effect of calcium, magnesium plays an important role in neuromuscular contraction. It also helps to regulate the acid-alkaline balance in the body.

Magnesium helps to promote the absorption and metabolism of other minerals, as well as the utilization of the B-vitamins and vitamins C and E. It aids during bone growth and is necessary for the proper functioning of the nerves and muscles.

Magnesium has been shown to be protective to DNA as the mineral is vital to telomerase activity. Telomerase is the enzyme responsible for telomere lengthening, a phenomenon associated with longevity and cell vitality.

Magnesium is widely distributed in food sources, but is found chiefly in fresh green vegetables, where it is an essential element of chlorophyll. Other excellent sources are un-milled raw wheat germ, soybeans, figs, corn, apples, and oil-rich seeds and nuts, especially almonds. Dolomite, a natural dietary supplement, is also rich in magnesium.

Evidence suggests that the balance between calcium and magnesium is especially important. If calcium consumption is high, magnesium intake must also be high. The magnesium requirement is further influenced by the amounts of protein, phosphorus, and vitamin D in the diet. The need is also increased when the blood-cholesterol level is high or the consumption of protein is high. Magnesium oxide is preferred over dolomite. When dolomite is taken, additional supplementation with hydrochloric acid is needed to ensure that the dolomite is dissolved properly. Because magnesium acts as an alkali, it should not be taken after meals.

It is estimated that the typical American diet provides only about 120 milligrams. Large amounts of magnesium can be toxic, especially if the calcium intake is low and the phosphorus intake is high. Excessive magnesium is usually excreted adequately, but in the event of kidney failure, there is a greater danger of toxicity because the rate of excretion is much lower.

Magnesium deficiency can occur in patients who have diabetes, pancreatitis, or kidney malfunction; are alcoholic or consume a high-carbohydrate diet. A deficiency is related to coronary heart disease, since it results in the formation of clots in the heart and brain, and may contribute to calcium deposits. The symptoms include apprehensiveness, muscle twitching, tremors, confusion, and disorientation. Also, magnesium deficiency may be an initiating factor in the evolution of endothelial dysfunction. Dysfunction in the endothelium is part of the disease process that can lead to the development of atherosclerosis.

## MANGANESE

Manganese is needed for healthy skin, bone, and cartilage formation, as well as glucose tolerance. It also helps activate superoxide dismutase (SOD)—an important antioxidant enzyme. Inadequate manganese levels increase mitochondrial oxidants and subsequent mitochondrial decay. Low levels of manganese can be associated with impaired glucose tolerance, as well as altered carbohydrate and lipid metabolism.

Many people consume less than the 2.5–5 mg of manganese currently considered safe and adequate. Nonetheless, clear deficiencies are rare. Individuals with osteoporosis sometimes have low blood levels of manganese, suggestive of deficiency. Manganese is found in nuts, wheat germ, wheat bran, leafy green vegetables, beet tops, pineapple, and seeds.

Whether most people would benefit from manganese supplementation remains unclear. Amounts found in supplements (5–20 mg) have not been linked with any toxicity. Excessive intake of manganese can lead to the rare side effects of dementia and psychiatric symptoms. Preliminary research suggests that individuals with cirrhosis may not be able to properly excrete manganese; until more is known, these people should not supplement manganese. Several minerals, such as calcium reduce the absorption of manganese. Zinc and copper work together with manganese to activate superoxide dismutase, now called SOD2 (or MnSOD).

## SELENIUM

Selenium is an essential mineral found in minute amounts in the body. It works closely with vitamin E in some of its metabolic actions, and in the promotion of normal body growth and fertility. Selenium is a natural antioxidant and appears to preserve the elasticity of tissue by delaying the oxidation of polyunsaturated fatty acids, which can cause solidification of tissue proteins.

Selenium is found in the bran and germ of cereals; in vegetables such as broccoli, onion, and tomatoes and in tuna. The liver and kidneys contain four to five times as much selenium as do the muscles and other tissues. Selenium is normally excreted in the urine. Its presence in the feces is an indication of improper absorption.

The RDA for selenium for adults is extremely minute—five to ten parts of selenium per one million parts of food or other minerals is considered toxic. This is due to the tendency of selenium to replace sulfur in biological compounds and to inhibit the action of some enzymes. Selenium can be toxic in its pure form, so supplements should be taken with care. Reported instances of toxicity have occurred in areas where the selenium content of the soil is high. And while low doses of selenium are considered useful in preventing cataracts, higher doses have actually been found to induce a cataract. Several reports have shown selenium deficiency causes defects in mitochondrial structure, integrity, and electron transport chain function. An increased risk of cancer and decreased immune system function has been associated with selenium deficiency.

A deficiency of selenium may encourage premature aging. This is because selenium preserves tissue elasticity. This is of major significance for the crystalline lens, which becomes less flexible with age.

## SODIUM

Sodium is an essential mineral found predominantly in the extracellular fluids such as the vascular fluids within the blood vessels and the interstitial fluids surrounding the cells. The remaining sodium in the body is found within the bones.

Sodium functions with potassium to equalize the acid-alkaline balance in the blood. Along with potassium, it helps to regulate the water balance within the body—that is, it helps to control the distribution of fluids on either side of the cell walls. Sodium and potassium are also involved in muscle contraction and expansion, and in nerve stimulation. Another important function of sodium is keeping the other blood minerals soluble so that they will not build up into deposits in the bloodstream. It helps to purge carbon dioxide from the body, aids digestion, and functions in the production of hydrochloric acid in the stomach. In addition, it acts with chlorine to improve blood and lymph health.

Sodium is found in virtually all foods, especially in sodium chloride (table salt). High concentrations are found in seafood, carrots, beets, poultry, and meat. Kelp is an excellent supplemental source of sodium.

There is no established dietary requirement for sodium, but it is generally observed that the usual intake far exceeds the need. The average

American ingests 3 to 7 grams of sodium and 6 to 18 grams of sodium chloride each day. The NRC recommends a daily sodium-chloride intake of 1 gram for every 1 kilogram (35 ounces) of water consumed.

An excess of sodium in the diet may cause potassium to be lost in the urine. Abnormal fluid retention accompanied by dizziness and swelling of the legs or face can also occur. Diets containing excessive amounts of sodium contribute to an increase in blood pressure. The simplest way to reduce sodium intake is to eliminate table salt and reduce bread in the diet. Yes, bread is the second largest contributor of sodium in the diet.

## ZINC

Zinc is an essential trace mineral that occurs in the body in a larger amount than any other trace element except iron. The human body contains approximately 1.8 grams of zinc, compared to nearly 5.0 grams of iron.

Zinc has a variety of functions. It is related to the normal absorption and action of the vitamins, especially vitamin A and the B complex. It is a constituent of at least twenty-five of the enzymes involved in digestion and metabolism. It is a component of insulin, and part of the enzyme that is needed to break down alcohol. It also functions in carbohydrate digestion and phosphorus metabolism. It has an important role in general growth and development, the function of the prostate gland, the healing of wounds and burns, and the synthesis of DNA.

Zinc, like magnesium, is a powerful anti-inflammatory mineral, although it is known primarily for its role in improving the function and performance of the immune system. Zinc becomes more important as we age, since immune dysfunction and inflammation become more pronounced and problematic with age.

Low zinc intakes are common, as 10% of the US population ingest under 50% of the RDA. Zinc deficiency in human cells in culture causes marked release of oxidants resulting in significant oxidative damage to DNA. Zinc deficiency is also associated with cancer.

The best sources of all the trace elements in proper balance are natural unprocessed foods- especially those grown in organically enriched soil. Diets high in protein, whole-grain products, brewer's yeast, wheat bran, wheat germ, and pumpkin seeds are usually high in zinc.

Zinc is relatively nontoxic, although poisoning may result from eating a food that has been stored in a galvanized container. High intakes of zinc interfere with copper utilization, causing incomplete iron metabolism. When zinc is added to the diet, vitamin A is also needed in larger amounts.

Many supplements (including the AREDS formulas) use the zinc oxide form to incorporate into their formulas. However, this is the least biologically active form of zinc and it must be combined with the proper balance of copper to avoid severe reaction. Monomethionine zinc is the most bioavailable form of zinc and the only form that does not interfere with copper absorption.

## ANTIOXIDANTS

All the vitamins and minerals that are antioxidants operate in a similar manner in the body. They play an important role in the body's basic defense system against disease, infection, premature aging, and, possibly, the adverse effects of strenuous athletic performance. Here is some background on how the antioxidants work.

At the root of many diseases and the aging process are a group of highly reactive substances called free radicals or oxidants (also referred to as Reactive Oxygen Species, or ROS). These chemical compounds consist of two or more elements bound together by a chemical bond, with an unpaired, or "extra," electron. The unpaired electron makes the free radical very reactive and unstable. To stabilize itself, a free radical seeks out and grabs an electron from a stable compound. This, in turn, creates a new free radical. A chain reaction is begun, thus extending the damage of even a small number of these reactive compounds.

Once in the body, free radicals attack cell components and cause damage to cells and tissues in the body. Common sites of attack are the polyunsaturated fatty acids in cell membranes. This free radical-induced damage alters the cell membrane structure and function. The membrane is no longer able to transport nutrients, oxygen, or water into the cell, or to regulate the removal of waste products. Continued free radical attack ruptures the cell membrane, causing the loss of the cellular components and rendering the cell useless. The intracellular chemicals leak into and damage the surrounding tissues. This process is associated with the initiation of numerous disorders from arthritis to cardiovascular disease.

Free radical damage to tissues or molecules might be an initiating factor of atherosclerosis. Oxidative damage to the arteries attracts platelets, while the damaged artery becomes a place for cholesterol to accumulate. Oxidized cholesterol (LDLs) might contribute to the process and increase adhesion at the site of the injury. Free radicals also damage the cells' mitochondria, which results in limited or halted production of energy for all the cell processes. Free radical damage to enzymes and other proteins limits the building of body tissues and causes the accumulation of protein fragments. Both of these conditions are noted in the premature aging of tissues. Finally, a cell cannot reproduce normally when its genetic code has been altered by free radicals. At best, the cell dies. At worst, the cell mutates into a cancerous cell.

Free radicals are unavoidable. They are formed during the normal metabolic process. They also are obtained from some foods, inhaled with polluted air and tobacco smoke, and generated in the environment by radiation and herbicides. Fortunately, the body has an anti-free radical system composed of antioxidant enzymes such as superoxide dismutase (SOD) and glutathione peroxidase; vitamins such as C, E, and beta-carotene; minerals such as zinc and selenium;

herbs such as bilberry and ginkgo; and other nutrients such as cysteine, pine bark extract, coenzyme Q10, and the bioflavonoids. These antioxidants intercede, deactivating the free radicals and rendering them harmless before they can cause irreversible damage to the body's tissues. They are currently being thoroughly investigated for their role in the prevention of many major diseases, including eye diseases such as cataracts and AMD.

## OTHER HELPFUL NUTRIENTS

### Phytochemicals

Phytochemicals are defined as bioactive nutrient plant chemicals that may provide desirable health benefits beyond basic nutrition to reduce the risk of major chronic diseases. The action of phytochemicals varies by color and type of the food.

They may act as antioxidants, hormones, enzyme stimulators, antibacterials or nutrient protectors, or prevent carcinogens from forming.

Sources of phytochemical are brightly colored fruits: berries, pears, tomatoes, cantaloupe, apricot, apples. Some of the more significant vegetables are broccoli, turnips, celery, carrots, spinach, kale, Bok choy, cabbage, olives, and Brussels sprouts. Also, whole grains, cereal, beans, lentils, soy nuts and seeds. Other plant foods include red wine, green tea, and garlic. There is no recommended dietary allowance for phytochemicals.

There are four general categories of phytochemicals: Carotenoids, Polyphenols, Organosulfur and Alkaloids. We will review the specific nutrient categories that have shown positive effects on the eyes and visual system.

### Carotenoids

This section is so important that it is covered again in the later chapters of this book.

Carotenoids in general are yellow, orange, or red pigments that are soluble in lipids. There are several sub-classifications of carotenoids, but the one most familiar are the pro-vitamin A carotenoids and the non-pro-vitamin A carotenoids, those that can and cannot be converted to vitamin A in the body. All consist of 40 carbons and contain a long linear polyene chain made of carbons connecting by alternating double bonds. To date, over 600 carotenoids have been identified in nature, but are only produced by plants, algae and bacteria. Animals appear to be incapable of biosynthesizing carotenoids, but all kinds of animals use them for a variety of purposes including coloration, and therefore they must obtain carotenoids from their diet. In humans it has been identified that about 40-50 are consumed typically in the diet but only 14 have been detected in serum. Only two of these have been found in the retina: lutein and zeaxanthin. A third carotenoid, meso-zeaxanthin is also found in the central retina but not routinely taken in the diet. (see below)

## Lutein

The lutein (LOO-teen), zeaxanthin and meso-zeaxanthin present together in the macula are known as macular pigment. Macular pigment appears as a yellow tint. The intense deposition of the yellow pigments in and around the fovea provided the basis for the clinical description of this area as the macula lutea or yellow spot. Macular pigment, likely via its blue light filtering property, has been shown in a number of clinical trials to enhance visual performance – the ability to perceive detailing carryout visual tasks. High levels of macular pigment contribute to improved visual acuity, glare tolerance and recovery, contrast sensitivity, chromatic aberration and photophobia in healthy individuals as well as those diagnosed with age-related eye diseases. Improvements in these parameters of visual performance can have a major impact on everyday activities. In other words, lutein and zeaxanthin act like "internal sunglasses" for the eyes.

Lutein and zeaxanthin are found naturally together in vegetables such as spinach, kale, broccoli, corn, green peas and green beans as well as other foods such as eggs. The bioavailability of lutein, unlike that of many other nutrients, is enhanced by chopping and cooking the food. This is likely due to the disruption of the strong interaction between chlorophyll and lutein molecules. It is difficult however, to obtain beneficial amounts of lutein and zeaxanthin from diet alone. Interventional studies report that 10 mg of lutein per day is effective in improving vision and reducing the risk of certain eye conditions. A survey of the standard American diet showed an approximate daily intake of 2 mg of lutein.

The ability of the macular pigment to absorb or filter blue light is measured as macular pigment optical density (MPOD). MPOD is an optical indicator of the concentration of lutein and zeaxanthin in the macula is becoming an accepted biomarker not only for predicting the risk for disease but also for visual function. In numerous studies MPOD is linearly related to the levels of lutein in the serum and positively correlated with dietary intake of lutein and zeaxanthin. MPOD measurement is a relatively new technology with only a few devices commercially available to evaluate it; however, it has been well studied clinically. Dozens of studies have been published demonstrating an increased macular pigment following lutein and/or zeaxanthin supplementation at a range of 2 to 30 mg per day or a high carotenoid diet. The degree of increase in MPOD levels following lutein or zeaxanthin supplementation varies, likely due to subject demographics, disease state, measurement method, diet, BMI, supplementation regimen or other factors.

There is a growing body of evidence, although not conclusive, that supports that low levels of MPOD may be a risk factor for certain age-related eye conditions. Increased levels in MPOD may provide greater protection against oxidative damage, which contributes in part to the manifestation of AMD. For example, risk factors for AMD including tobacco use, light iris color, advanced age, obesity, and female gender are associated with low levels of MPOD. Significantly less macular pigment has been found in eyes at high risk for AMD because of advanced disease in the fellow eye compared with eyes with no known risk.

SR-B1 has recently been identified as a lutein binding protein in the retina, and this same receptor plays a role in the selective uptake in the gut.

In the blood, lutein is transported via high-density lipoproteins (HDL). Genes controlling SR-B1 and HDL levels predispose to AMD, which supports the involvement of cholesterol/lutein transport pathways. Apart from beneficial effects of lutein intake on various visual function tests, recent findings show that lutein can affect immune responses and inflammation. Lutein diminishes the expression of various ocular inflammation models including endotoxin induced uveitis, laser induced choroidal neovascularization, streptozotocin induced diabetes and experimental retinal ischemia and reperfusion. In vitro studies show that lutein suppresses NF kappa-B activation as well as the expression of iNOS and COX-2. Since AMD has features of a chronic low-grade systemic inflammatory response, attention to the exact role of lutein in this disease has shifted from a local effect in the eye towards a possible systemic anti-inflammatory function.

In addition to being present in the macula, lutein is also deposited in the glands, albeit at much lower concentrations. The fact that oxidation of the lens is the major cause of cataracts suggest that antioxidant nutrients may play a role in cataract prevention. In support of this hypothesis, lutein and zeaxanthin intake from dietary sources has been linked to the reduction in risk for cataract extraction in a number of epidemiologic studies.

Nutritional intervention has also been shown to slow visual field loss associated with retinitis pigmentosa. The National Eye Institute recommends that most adult patients with the common forms of retinitis pigmentosa take a supplement of 15,000 IU of vitamin A daily under the supervision of their eyecare professional. A study published in April 2010 suggests that the addition of 12 mg per day of lutein to this vitamin A regimen can slow the loss of mid-peripheral field sensitivity to a greater degree than vitamin A alone.

MPOD has the potential to become a commonly tested biomarker to measure an individual's risk for eye disease and to assess visual function knowledge of individuals MPOD level indicates whether he or she is getting enough lutein and zeaxanthin through their diet or supplementation regimen. Identification of individuals at low, medium and high risk for eye disease can be made based on their MPOD level. MPOD is typically measured on a logarithmic scale and values range from undetectable to over 1.0 optical density units (d.u.). Experts agree that the central MPOD below 0.2d.u. is considered low, between 0.2 and 0.5d.u. is midrange and levels above 0.5d.u. are high. Commercial MPOD measuring instrumentation is available throughout the industry.

## Zeaxanthin

As often mentioned in the previous section, lutein and zeaxanthin (zee-ah-ZAN-thin) are often mentioned together. This is due to the very similar chemical structure of the two molecules. Zeaxanthin is one of the most common carotenoid alcohols found in nature. It is the pigment that gives paprika (made from bell peppers), corn, saffron, and many other plants their characteristic color. Spirulina is also a rich source and can serve as a dietary supplement. Zeaxanthin breaks down to form picrocrocin and safranal, which are responsible for the taste and aroma of saffron.

Zeaxanthin's role is to help protect the eye from the high-energy, blue-wave light. Zeaxanthin also protects the ganglion cells and helps the eye repair itself. In fact, studies have shown that the portion of the macula with the highest concentration of zeaxanthin is the last to degenerate. The highest density of zeaxanthin is at the very center of the macula, thus affording it the greatest protection, whereas in the peripheral retina, lutein predominates. Although there is no recommended daily intake level for zeaxanthin, a recommended amount is 8mg daily for anyone diagnosed with macular degeneration and 2-4 mg for those taking it as a preventative measure.

Several observational studies have connected high dietary intake of foods providing zeaxanthin with lower incidence of AMD. There is currently insufficient evidence to assess the effectiveness of dietary or supplemental antioxidants in treatment or primary prevention of AMD, or the formation or progression of cataracts. Any benefit is more likely to be apparent in subpopulations of individuals exposed to high oxidative stress, such as heavy smokers or those with poor nutrition.

## Meso-zeaxanthin

A third macular pigment called meso-zeaxanthin (MEEZO-zee-ah-zan-thin) also contributes. Discovered at the Florida International University, meso-zeaxanthin is found in the retina but unlike lutein and zeaxanthin, has not been isolated from blood plasma or the liver, is not produced within the body nor derived from the traditional American diet.

Meso-zeaxanthin can only be absorbed through natural conversion of enzymes from lutein. It is a metabolite of lutein and concentrated along with zeaxanthin in the central macula. It is a powerful antioxidant, allowing greater blue light filtration as a damage preventing measure. In rare cases, there is poor conversion from lutein to meso-zeaxanthin. For these patients, supplementation of meso-zeaxanthin directly fortifies pigment density in the central macula without known adverse side-effects. Due to its biochemical properties, all supplements of meso-zeaxanthin must be combined with lutein and zeaxanthin. In many supplement formula labels, meso-zeaxanthin is referred to as "zeaxanthin isomers".

Supplementation with meso-zeaxanthin is controversial due to potential carotenoid competition. Dietary lutein and zeaxanthin have emerged as crucial, if not essential, brain nutrients. More work needs to be done addressing the issue of carotenoid competition.

Meso-zeaxanthin was not included in the AREDS or AREDS2 studies. Given that it is not readily found in the diet, the supplementation of this carotenoid is speculative. It is found in shrimp shells, turtle skin and fish skin- all in small amounts. It is only found in eggs of chickens that have been fed meso-zeaxanthin in the feed.

## OTHER CAROTENOIDS OF NOTE

### *Beta-Carotene*

Beta-carotene is a carotenoid, a class of compounds related to vitamin A. Some carotenoids, such as beta-carotene, can act as precursors of vitamin A. When a food or supplement containing beta-carotene is consumed, the beta-carotene is converted into vitamin A in the liver. According to recent reports, beta-carotene appears to aid in cancer prevention by scavenging, or neutralizing, free radicals. However, it should be noted that there is no beta-carotene, per se, in the eye. We will review all of the important eye-related carotenoids later on in this section.

Once converted into vitamin A, carotene is absorbed the same way as preformed vitamin A. The conversion of carotene into vitamin A is never 100 percent complete. Approximately one-third of the carotene in food is converted into vitamin A. Less than one-fourth of the carotene in carrots and root vegetables undergoes conversion, and about one-half of the carotene in leafy green vegetables does. Some unchanged carotene is absorbed into the circulatory system and stored in the fat tissues rather than in the liver. Unabsorbed carotene is excreted.

The degree to which carotene is utilized by the body varies with the food source and the way the food is prepared. Cooking, puréeing, and mashing of a vegetable rupture the cell membranes and therefore make the carotene more available for absorption. Factors interfering with the absorption of vitamin A and carotene include strenuous physical activity performed within four hours of consumption of the nutrient, intake of mineral oil, excessive consumption of alcohol, excessive consumption of iron, and the use of cortisone and other medications. The intake of polyunsaturated fatty acids with carotene results in rapid destruction of the carotene unless antioxidants also are present. Even cold weather can hinder the transport and metabolism of vitamin A and carotene. Diabetics cannot convert carotene to vitamin A

Supplemental beta-carotene was shown to increase the risk of lung cancer in smokers in a poorly designed Finnish, Alpha-Tocopherol, Beta-Carotene Cancer Prevention (ATBC) study. A second study, Carotenoid and Retinol Efficacy Trial (CARET) also found a higher incidence of lung cancer in those people taking a whopping 30 mg of synthetic beta-carotene, plus 25,000 IU of preformed Vitamin A retinol.

The amount of supplemental Vitamin A and beta-carotene included in both the ATBC and CARET studies was far beyond the safe upper limits (UL) for daily consumption established by the Food and Nutrition Board at The Institute of Medicine. The UL established by The Institute of Medicine for the combination of preformed Vitamin A as retinol, and pre-formed Vitamin A as retinol activity carotenoids (primarily beta-carotene) is 10,000 IU or approximately 3,000 retinol equivalents (RAE) per day.

At about the same time, the 12-year long Physicians' Health Study (PHS), involving more than 22,000 physician volunteers, showed no statistical increase in lung cancer rates in doctors who were taking a full-spectrum multiple and 50 mg of synthetic beta carotene—even in the 11% of physician volunteers who were heavy smokers.

The American Journal of Epidemiology data clearly suggests that, in fact, smokers who consume small amounts of natural supplemental beta-carotene in combination with a wide variety of supplemental anti-oxidants actually have an overall 16% lower risk of developing lung and other cancer. Beta-carotene is not vitamin A. It is a rate-limiting pre-formed vitamin A hydrocarbon carotenoid. It competes with the xanthophyll carotenoids, lutein and zeaxanthin (see below), for cellular transport space, therefore excessive amounts of supplemental beta-carotene are not recommended to vision patients for that reason, as well. The body's need for Vitamin A is so critical it will convert plant-based hydrocarbon beta-carotene to Vitamin A retinol, if and when the retinol liver stores are deficient. If there is no Vitamin A retinol deficiency, beta-carotene functions as a powerhouse antioxidant, particularly against retina-damaging singlet oxygen, and does not convert to retinol. The beta carotene/retinol conversion also becomes less efficient with the aging process; so research-focused nutritional biochemists stopped recommending beta-carotene as a sole source of supplemental Vitamin A for older men and women years ago.

### *Lycopene*

Carotenoids like lycopene are important pigments found in photosynthetic pigment-protein complexes in plants, photosynthetic bacteria, fungi, and algae. They are responsible for the bright colors of fruits and vegetables, perform various functions in photosynthesis, and protect photosynthetic organisms from excessive light damage.

Lycopene is a key intermediate in the biosynthesis of many important carotenoids, such as beta-carotene and xanthophylls. Given this connection to beta-carotene and xanthophylls, many sources maintain that it is critical to eye health. However, lycopene is not modified to vitamin A in the body so it can be accessible for other benefits such as antioxidation. There is no lycopene found in the eye and any positive effect of this carotenoid to ocular health is secondary.

### *Astaxanthin*

Astaxanthin is a unique carotenoid that is ubiquitous in marine ecosystems. Originating in aquatic microorganisms and microalgae, astaxanthin naturally accumulates in the food chain to lend red and pink coloration to higher organisms such as krill, shrimp and salmon. Among carotenoids, astaxanthin is distinguished by a unique chemical structure, two extra hydroxyl groups. This physical nuance affords a tenfold greater antioxidant capacity than beta-carotene and lutein.

In addition to its well-established antioxidant potency, astaxanthin maintains inflammatory balance activity by modulating a central intracellular switch known as nuclear factor kappa B (NfkB). Through regulating gene expression, NFkB controls the inflammatory response in almost every cell, including those comprising the immune system, connective tissue, vascular chair, adipose tissue, eyes and skin. Accordingly, the effect of support for information with astaxanthin has been documented in clinical research.

While some references point to the positive effects of astaxanthin on ocular tissue, the emerging science on this aspect of the carotenoid is still yet to be determined. There is no astaxanthin normally residing within the structure of the eye itself. However, it does have that positive effect on striated muscle and there are six striated muscles controlling each eyeball. Thus, a powerful antioxidant that relieves muscle stress in the extraocular muscles might have an effect on the functioning of the visual system. The exact effects of astaxanthin on eye health are yet to be resolved.

### *Capsanthin*

One of the more recently stabilized carotenoids is capsanthin from *Capsicum annum* or CCA. This is different than the herb Capsaicin. Capsaicin has been proposed to have anti-obesity effects via its ability to increase energy expenditure and lipid oxidation, attenuate postprandial insulin response, increase satiety, and reduce appetite and energy intake. Capsanthin, on the other hand, is a lipophilic carotenoid, majorly found in the pericarp of ripe red pepper (Capsicum spp). The greater light absorbing as well as antioxidant capacities of Capsanthin are due to the presence of eleven conjugated double bonds, a conjugated keto group, and a cyclopentane ring.

It was demonstrated that the oral administration of CapsiClear™ (the trade name for Capsanthin) in an animal study significantly reduced the intraocular pressure (IOP) in IOP elevated-induced rats in both eyes, even at a low dose of 20 mg/kg body weight. A beneficial effect was seen as early as ten days with treatment, and IOP returned to normal after 28 days, comparable to the vehicle-treated control groups. The IOP lowering effect of CapsiClear was similar to the effect obtained with the reference test drug, pilocarpine.

CapsiClear was found to be safe and well-tolerated and did not result in any clinical signs of toxicity, mortality, changes in body weight, and feed consumption at all tested dose levels. There were no treatment-related changes in histopathology, hematology, and clinical chemistry parameters. Levels of critical antioxidants, such as GSH and SOD in the plasma, remained unaffected by treatment with CapsiClear. Thus, oral administration of CapsiClear in IOP-induced rats has shown to be beneficial without any adverse effects.

In this same study, it was found that administration of CapsiClear showed clinical benefits by maintaining the integrity of the corneal surface and ameliorating surface inflammation in a BAC-induced DED (dry eye) rat model. CapsiClear has a noticeable therapeutic effect on some ocular symptoms such as IOP, tear break-time, tear production, corneal inflammation, and corneal repair. CCA supplementation reduced oxidative stress by increasing glutathione peroxidase (GPX), lactoferrin (LTF), and nitric oxide (NO) production. A non-toxic *Capsicum annum* (CCA) could also inhibit the expressions of inflammatory cytokines, tumor necrosis factor-alpha (TNF-α), interleukins (IL-2, IL-4, IL-6), and pro-inflammatory mediator, matrix metalloproteinase 9 (MMP9), vascular cell adhesion molecule 1 (VCAM1), and prostaglandin E2. This research demonstrated for the first time that oral administration of CapsiClear significantly ameliorated BAC-induced DED in a rodent model. The mechanism of therapeutic action might be related to its direct inhibition of TNF-α/ IL-2/ IL-4/ IL-6 as well as MMP9, VCAM1, and PTGS2 expression.

## The Polyphenols

Another category of phytochemical is called polyphenols. Phenols are a class of organic compounds that contain a hydroxyl group (-OH) bonded to an aromatic hydrocarbon group. Phenol ($C_6H_5OH$) is the simplest phenol. Phenols are found in plants, animals, and humans. They are also produced by the chemical industry; chlorinated phenols are almost entirely man-made. Phenolic compounds are classified as simple phenols or polyphenols based on the number of phenol units in the molecule.

There are four subcategories of polyphenols, which include bioflavonoids, phenolic acids, stilbenes, and lignans. Below is a description of the polyphenols related to eye health.

### *Bioflavonoids*

There are several classes of bioflavonoids:

- *Flavanols* are linked to many health benefits, including decreasing risk for heart disease. Some sources are lettuce, tomatoes, onions, apples, berries, and tea.
- *Isoflavones* are phytoestrogens, a form of estrogen in food.
- *Flavanones* are found in citrus fruits. They function as antioxidants, lower cholesterol, and reduce inflammation.

- *Anthocyanins* are the coloring in a wide variety of berries.
- *Chalcones* are thought to be antioxidants. Some are used in beauty products. Sources include tomatoes, pears, strawberries, and wheat.
- *Flavones* are found in herbs and spices such as thyme, oregano, celery, peppermint, and parsley.

The bioflavonoids are water-soluble and composed of a group of brightly colored substances that often appear in fruits and vegetables as companions to vitamin C. They were first discovered as substances in the white part, not the juice, of citrus fruits. The edible part of citrus fruits contains ten times more bioflavonoids than the strained juice.

The bioflavonoids are essential for the proper absorption and use of vitamin C. They assist vitamin C in keeping the collagen in healthy condition. They also have the ability to increase the strength of the capillaries and to regulate the capillaries' permeability. These actions help to prevent hemorrhages and ruptures in the capillaries and connective tissue, and to build a protective barrier against infections. Retinal hemorrhages may be reduced to some degree by the use of a vitamin C-bioflavonoid combination.

Although flavonoids can be ingested as supplements, it is best to get them from food.

- *Berries* contain flavonoids, with the greatest concentration in blackberries. Blueberries, cherries, and raspberries contain all the subclasses of flavonoids. Strawberries contain moderate amounts of the subclass anthocyanins.
- *Red cabbage* is another reliable source of anthocyanins. These flavonoids have protective effects against cancer, cardiovascular disease, diabetes, and age-related cognitive disorders.
- *Onions* are basic to many native cuisines and are full of nutrients, including flavanols, which can reduce the risk of prostate cancer.
- *Kale* is also a useful source of flavanols. It's a good base for salads, soups and stews, smoothies, and protein shakes.

- *Parsley* contains more than 130 milligrams of flavanols per gram, more than any other food in the American diet. It's often added to soups and sauces or sprinkled over food and used as a garnish.
- *Tea*, as a hot or cold drink, is an effortless way to add flavonoids to the diet. These include black, green, and oolong teas, good for both heart and brain health.
- *Red wine* is a reliable source of flavanols. It remains, however, a controversial element of diet. Some studies showed potential benefits of one glass of wine per day on decreasing heart disease, but it increases the risk for cancer.
- *Dark chocolate and cocoa* are both high in flavanols. In particular, cocoa has been studied for its protective effect on the cardiovascular system and for boosting cognitive function. However, moderation should be taken with chocolate since it contains large amounts of sugar.
- *Citrus fruits* contain flavanones. Using their juice will concentrate the compounds. You may like lemon or lime juice added to hot or ice water.
- *Soybeans* are one of the best sources of isoflavones. They can be eaten as tofu, tempeh, and edamame. They are believed to help protect against reproductive cancers such as breast, ovarian, prostate, and testicular cancers.

The absorption and storage properties, daily requirements, deficiency symptoms, and body utilization of the bioflavonoids are all similar to those of vitamin C.

### *Phenolic Acids*

Phenolic acids are phenolic compounds and types of aromatic acid compounds. Phenolic acids can be found in many plant species. Their content in dried fruits can be high. They can also be found in several mushroom species. They are also a part of the humic substances, which are the major organic constituents of soil humus.

Phenolic acids act as signaling molecules in plant-microbe interactions. They can act as agents in plant defense. They have a role in a wide range of biological and pharmacological properties. Phenols are commonly found in curcumin (turmeric root), gallic acid (garlic), coumaric acid (coumadin) and caffeic acid (coffee). All of these molecules have numerous health benefits, including anti-inflammatory, antioxidant, cardioprotective, and more.

### *Stilbenes*

The most well-known stilbene is resveratrol. Resveratrol is a chemical mostly found in red grapes and products made from these grapes (wine, juice). It may be helpful for hay fever and weight loss. Due to its multiple biological properties, resveratrol could help fight the main molecular events of ocular pathologies through its antioxidant power, as well as its anti-inflammatory and anti-angiogenic properties. Sources include Japanese knotweed and red wine.

Resveratrol might have many effects in the body, including expanding blood vessels and reducing blood clotting. It may also decrease pain and swelling, reduce levels of sugar in the blood, and help the body fight against disease. People often consume resveratrol in small amounts in foods. However, the amount of resveratrol in red wine would require drinking about 14 glasses of wine per day, so obviously not the recommended mode of intake. Resveratrol supplements are possibly safe when taken by mouth in doses up to 1500 mg daily for up to 3 months. Higher doses of up to 2000-3000 mg daily have been used safely for 2-6 months. But these higher doses are more likely to cause stomach upset.

Resveratrol is most commonly used for high cholesterol, cancer, heart disease, and many other conditions. Regarding eye-related concerns, the literature reports that resveratrol is able to act on various cell types of the eye by increasing the level of natural antioxidant enzymatic and molecular defenses. Resveratrol anti-inflammatory effects are due to its capacity to limit the expression of pro-inflammatory factors, such as interleukins and prostaglandins, and also to decrease the chemo-attraction and recruitment of immune cells to the inflammatory site. In addition to this, resveratrol was shown to possess anti-VEGF effects and to inhibit the proliferation and migration of vascular endothelial cells, which is significant for AMD patients. Resveratrol has the potential to be used in a range of human ocular diseases and conditions.

One product that uses resveratrol is called Longevinex®. Longevinex® is a low dose over-the-counter oral resveratrol-based matrix of red wine solids, vitamin D3 and inositol hexaphosphate (IP6) with established bioavailability, safety, and short-term efficacy against the earliest signs of human atherosclerosis, murine cardiac reperfusion injury, clinical retinal neovascularization, and stem cell survival. It has been previously reported to improve short-term findings for dry and wet age-related macular degeneration patients.

### *Acetyl-L-Carnitine (ALC)*

ALC is a delivery form for the amino acid, L-carnitine. It transports Omega-3 long-chain fatty acids across the mitochondrial membranes into the mitochondria and transports small-chain and medium-chain fatty acids out of the mitochondria in order to maintain normal Co-enzyme A levels in these organelles within the cell. This is particularly important for maintenance of retina health due to the large number of mitochondria within retinal cells.

Acetyl-L-carnitine levels may decrease with advancing age. However, because it is not an essential nutrient, true deficiencies do not occur. Most research involving acetyl-L-carnitine has used 500 mg three times per day, though some research has used double this amount.

Side effects from taking acetyl-L-carnitine are uncommon, although skin rash, increased appetite, nausea, vomiting, agitation, and body odor have been reported in people taking excessive amounts of acetyl-L-carnitine.

### *Coenzyme Q10 (CoQ10)*

CoQ10 is a fat-soluble compound primarily synthesized by the body and also consumed in the diet. It is required for mitochondrial energy synthesis; thus, it is found in highest concentration in the inner membrane of the mitochondria. The primary function of CoQ10 is as a catalyst for metabolism. It also functions as an antioxidant in cell membranes and lipoproteins. Acting in conjunction with enzymes, CoQ10 speeds up the vital metabolic process, providing the energy that the cells need to digest food, heal wounds, maintain healthy muscles, and perform countless other bodily functions.

Because of the nutrient's essential role in energy production, it's not surprising that it is found in every cell in the body. It is especially abundant in the energy-intensive cells of the heart and retina. In addition, coenzyme Q10 acts as an antioxidant, much like vitamins C and E, helping to neutralize the cell-damaging free radicals.

CoQ10 is a component of the electron transport chain and participates in aerobic cellular respiration, generating energy in the form of ATP. Ninety-five percent of the human body's energy is generated this way. Therefore, those organs with the highest energy requirements—such as the heart, liver, eyes and kidney—have the highest CoQ10 concentrations. There are three redox states of coenzyme Q10: fully oxidized (ubiquinone), semiquinone (ubisemiquinone), and fully reduced (ubiquinol). The capacity of this molecule to exist in a completely oxidized form and a completely reduced form enables it to perform its functions in the electron transport chain and as an antioxidant respectively.

CoQ10 may play a role in preventing cancer, heart attacks, and other diseases linked to free-radical damage. It's also used as a general energy enhancer and anti-aging supplement. Supplementation helps not only boost energy but also cognitive functions for an overall energy boost. Because levels of the compound diminish with age (and with certain diseases), some doctors recommend daily supplementation beginning about age 40.

Coenzyme Q10 shares a biosynthetic pathway with cholesterol. The synthesis of an intermediary precursor of coenzyme Q10, mevalonate, is inhibited by some beta blockers, blood pressure-lowering medication, and statins. Statins can reduce serum levels of coenzyme Q10 by up to 40%, therefore CoQ10 supplements should be routinely taken with all statin drugs.

### *Hyaluronic Acid*

Hyaluronic acid (HA) is an anionic, non-sulfated glycosaminoglycan distributed widely throughout connective, epithelial, and neural tissues. It is approved for use in eye surgery (i.e., corneal transplantation, cataract surgery, glaucoma surgery, and to repair retinal detachment). HA binds cells together, lubricates joints, and helps maintain the shape of the eyeballs. HA is responsible for strength and integrity of scleral collagen, thus might be considered in the regimen for preventing or reducing myopia development or progression.

Hyaluronic acid is very good at retaining water. A quarter-teaspoon of hyaluronic acid holds about one and a half gallons of water. That's why hyaluronic acid is often used for treating dry eyes. Commercial eye drops with sodium hyaluronate are a good option for helping relieve dry eye symptoms, with options available without a prescription for even severe symptoms. HA can also help with irritation from prolonged exposure to sunlight, exposure to an air-conditioned or any dry environment.

### *Lactoferrin*

Lactoferrin is an anti-viral, anti-bacterial iron-binding glycoprotein that is particularly vital to tear production. It is also a mucous-specific anti-inflammatory molecule. Serum lactoferrin is produced by acinar cells in the lacrimal gland and possibly also from tear neutrophils during infection and inflammation. By binding iron, lactoferrin prevents the pathogen from obtaining sufficient iron, which it relies upon for growth.

The name comes from two root words: "lacto", referring to milk (and specifically "first milk" from lactation) and "ferrin", referring to its iron-binding nature. Due to its action in mucosal tissue, lactoferrin in tear fluid has been shown to be decreased in dry eye diseases such as Sjögren's syndrome. Lactoferrin was found to be negatively correlated to Rose Bengal staining, indicating that reduced lactoferrin was a marker of ocular surface damage. However, in evaporative dry eye in the absence of epithelial defects, tear lactoferrin was also found to be reduced.

Lactoferrin should be included in any oral supplement that addresses dry eye disease. A typical effective dosage would be 20 mg per day.

### *Pycnogenol*

Pycnogenol is a compound of natural chemicals. It comes from the bark of a European pine tree. It is thought to be an antioxidant that helps protect cells from damage.

Pycnogenol is the registered trademark name for a French formula. The active ingredients in pycnogenol can also be extracted from other sources, including peanut skin, grape seed, and witch hazel bark.

Pycnogenol has been shown to be effective in several disorders, including asthma, attention deficit hyperactivity disorder, chronic venous insufficiency, erectile dysfunction, hypertension, and osteoarthritis.

The commercial product is called Mirtogenol. Mirtogenol tablets contain 40mg of Pycnogenol, French maritime pine bark extract and 80mg of Mirtoselect®, standardized bilberry extract. Studies show a reduction in IOP was only about 3 mm Hg (25.2 to 22.2: not significant). However, an improved ocular blood flow may contribute to the prevention of glaucoma. The results of this study indicate that Mirtogenol may represent a safe preventative intervention for lowering the risk for developing symptomatic glaucoma by controlling IOP and improving ocular blood flow. A subsequent study showed that the improvements in retinal microcirculation were statistically significant for all management groups, with a marginally more evident benefit when Mirtogenol is added to latanoprost in study treated patients.

### *Pyrroloquinoline Quinone (PQQ)*

PQQ is a cofactor for bacterial redox reactions and is a signaling agent for proteins kinases involved in differentiation of mammalian cells. Rat studies show impressive efficacy for PQQ in stimulating mitochondrial biogenesis. Since mammalian cells cannot synthesize PQQ researchers believe the PQQ found in human tissue is likely derived from the diet as well as originating from enteric bacterial production.

Much of the research on PQQ to date has been conducted in animals but there is a growing body of work supporting its use in humans with no evidence of acute side effects or overt toxicity from amounts as high as 60 mg per day. Oral PQQ supplementation does increase indicators of mitochondrial efficiency in healthy humans. More work needs to be done in investigating the efficacy of PQQ for conditions known to have underpinnings in mitochondrial dysfunction but evidence so far is quite compelling for PQQ's role in helping to reduce age-related oxidative stress and rejuvenating healthy mitochondria. In vivo studies in rats also show beneficial effects from dietary supplementation with PQQ (2mg PQQ/kg of food).

### *Anthocyanidins*

Water-soluble pigments that account, in part, for the red, purple and blue colors of fruits and flowers (as a function of pH). Mediate a detergent-like agitation of cell membranes and light-induced damage to the RPE cell. They have been shown to inhibit development of AMD as well as slow the aging process, protect against heart disease and tumors, prevent blood clots, and fight inflammation and allergies.

Anthocyanidins are found in red and blue fruits (such as raspberries and blueberries/bilberries) and deep-colored vegetables.

### *Epigallocatechin gallate (EGCG)*

A catechin is a type of natural phenol and antioxidant and is a part of the chemical family of flavonoids. EGCG – the most abundant catechin in tea – is being researched for its potential to affect human health and disease. EGCG is used in many dietary supplements.

Catechins and epicatechins are found in cocoa, which has one of the highest contents of catechins, followed by prune juice. They are diverse among foods from peaches to green tea and vinegar, as well as barley grain. Açaí oil contains a significant amount of catechins as well.

In the eye, they function as a treatment and prevention of ocular angiogenic diseases: AMD, diabetic retinopathy, and corneal neovascularization. They protect the crystalline lens epithelial cells from the mitochondria-mediated apoptosis; thus, possible cataract prevention. Neuroprotective function pattern-evoked ERGs increased in amplitude and have a positive influence in inner retinal function with early to moderately advanced glaucomatous damage. They ameliorate the negative effect of high glucose concentrations on the cell viability and apoptotic rate. May be attributed to the regulation of inflammatory cytokines in diabetic retinopathy.

### *Lipoic Acid*

Lipoic acid is both water and fat-soluble and is a vital cofactor for production of enzymes necessary for mitochondrial function. Alpha-lipoic acid (ALA) works together with other antioxidants such as vitamins C and E. It is important for growth, helps to prevent cell damage, and helps the body rid itself of harmful toxins.

Several studies suggest that treatment with ALA may help reduce pain, burning, itching, tingling, and numbness in people who have peripheral neuropathy caused by diabetes. Alpha-lipoic acid has been used for years for this purpose in Europe. Other studies have shown that ALA speeds the removal of glucose from the blood of people with diabetes and that this antioxidant may prevent kidney damage associated with diabetes in animals.

ALA may prove useful in the treatment of chronic hepatitis because it relieves stress on the liver and helps rid the body of toxins. There have been several case reports of use of ALA in combination with silymarin (milk thistle) and selenium (a substance with liver-protecting and antioxidant properties) to help treat hepatitis C.

Because ALA can pass easily into the brain, it has protective effects on brain and nerve tissue and shows promise as a treatment for stroke and other brain disorders involving free radical damage. Animals treated with ALA, for example, suffered less brain damage and had a four times greater survival rate after a stroke than the animals who did not receive this supplement. While animal studies are encouraging, more research is needed to understand whether this benefit applies to people as well.

Additional conditions for which ALA may prove useful include heart failure, HIV, cataracts, and glaucoma (due to anti-oxidant activity). More research is underway in these areas. Good food sources of alpha-lipoic acid include spinach, broccoli, beef, Brewer's yeast, and certain organ meats (such as the kidney and heart).

# EYE STRUCTURES AND NUTRIENTS

WHILE THERE IS NO SIMPLE STRUCTURE FOR WHICH NUTRIENTS SUPPORT any particular part of the eye, there are some nutrients that are more prominent in certain parts of the eye. This list is general and you should realize that all nutrients work together to support our visual system.

## EYE STRUCTURES AND SUPPORTIVE NUTRIENTS

While most nutrients have overall effects on a variety of structures and organs in the body, some nutrients play a special role in the visual system. Here is a listing of the various structures within the eye and which nutrients play an important role in ocular health.

| Eye Structure | Nutrients |
|---|---|
| Aqueous Humor | Glutathione, Vitamin C, Vitamin E |
| Cornea | CoQ10, Collagen, Hyaluronic Acid |
| Crystalline Lens | Glutathione, Lutein, Potassium, Vitamin C, Vitamin E, Zeaxanthin, Protein |
| Optic Nerve | Glutathione, Vitamin B2, Vitamin B12 |
| Photoreceptors | DHA, Vitamin A, Zinc |
| Retinal Pigmented Epithelium | NAD+, Selenium, Vitamin E |
| Retinal Nerve Layer | Glutathione, Hyaluronic Acid, Lutein, Zeaxanthin |
| Sclera | Vitamin C, Collagen, Hyaluronic Acid, Iron, Proline |
| Tear Film | Essential Fatty Acids, Lactoferrin, Vitamin A |
| Vitreous Humor | Antioxidants, Hyaluronic Acid, Selenium, Vitamin C, Water |

# PART II
# EYE DISORDERS

# INTRODUCTION

Here we will list some of the most common eye disorders that confront optometrists often on a daily basis. Each section will start with a short description of the disorder, followed by charts with nutritional, herbal, and homeopathic suggestions when appropriate. Note that these are suggestions to supplement any medical treatment of the disorder, not to replace it. Lastly, there will be suggestions to offer to patients on how to assist in the treatment process.

## ACCOMMODATIVE INSUFFICIENCY

Any loss of accommodative ability before the age of 40 is considered abnormal. This is most commonly seen in school-aged children who have difficulty focusing on their reading materials. This condition is called *accommodative insufficiency.*

Patients typically think of this as a loss of "strength" of the eye muscles to be able to focus properly. We do know that the accommodative and convergence systems are neurologically coordinated (as shown by the ACA ratio) so they are linked to our accommodative function. Thus, improving striated muscle function may have some positive effects on the accommodative output.

Accommodative insufficiency can also masquerade as accommodative spasm. If the ciliary muscle is over-taxed for an extended period of time, it may be put into a spasmodic state. If testing for accommodative effort, the spastic state can appear as an "insufficiency". Transient induced myopia (TIM) is also a potential manifestation of this condition.

## CONVENTIONAL TREATMENT

There are two procedures that should be considered for treating accommodative insufficiency. The first is the conventional method of near-point glasses; the second is vision therapy. Although vision therapy is considered to be much more than simply eye exercises, in this case techniques are used to enhance the functional abilities of the muscle pairs to work in conjunction with each other.

## NUTRITIONAL SUPPORT

Nutrients to address this condition are designed to support smooth and striated muscles as well as increase oxygen utilization. The chart below will show those nutrients best suited for this condition.

| NUTRITIONAL SUPPLEMENTS | | |
|---|---|---|
| **Supplement** | **Directions for Use** | **Comments** |
| Astaxanthin | 6 mg daily | Protects cell membrane components from oxidative stress and inflammation; supports muscle function |
| Calcium | 800-1000 mg daily (depending on age) | Should be balance with equal amount of phosphorus and magnesium |
| Magnesium | 300-400 mg daily (depending on age) | Relaxes muscles |
| Vitamin B2 | 75 mg daily | Good for the nerves, muscles, and fatigue |
| Vitamin C | 500 mg twice daily | Nourishes the lens |
| Vitamin E | 200 IU daily | An antioxidant. |

| HOMEOPATHIC REMEDIES | | |
|---|---|---|
| **Remedy** | **Directions for Use** | **Comments** |
| Cocculuc 6c | 3–4 pellets under the tongue 3–4 times daily. | Good for accommodative insufficiency associated with nausea. |

*continued*

| HOMEOPATHIC REMEDIES (*con't*) | | |
|---|---|---|
| **Remedy** | **Directions for Use** | **Comments** |
| Gelsemium sempervirens 6c | 3–4 pellets under the tongue 3–4 times daily. | Good for accommodative insufficiency associated with headache. |
| Natrum muriaticum 6c | 3–4 pellets under the tongue | Good for accommodative insufficiency associated with anger or irritability. |

## AGE-RELATED MACULAR DEGENERATION (AMD)

*See* Macular Degeneration.

## ARCUS SENILIS

The condition of arcus senilis most often develops during the later years, but it is not uncommon in middle age or even younger. In arcus senilis, an opaque white ring encircles the corneas' periphery, however there is a clear section of cornea between the edge of the ring and the sclera. This is thought to be due either to the deposition of fat granules in the cornea or to hyaline degeneration. Hyaline degeneration is a type of tissue degeneration that results in rounded masses or broad bands of translucent tissue (like the cornea). It most often occurs in black patients about a decade earlier than white patients.

Arcus senilis generally is not considered to be of pathological importance, but from a biochemical viewpoint, it represents a specific metabolic disturbance and is possibly an indication of fat and cholesterol metabolism. The physiology, obviously disturbed, is not obvious here. According to some authorities, the condition is a known biometric indicator of biologic aging and mortality, especially in males.

Arcus is often associated with a vitamin D and magnesium deficiencies. The general consensus is that arcus senilis is normal in older adults, but can be a sign of elevated cholesterol in middle-aged or younger individuals. In younger (30's-40's) individuals, a lipid blood panel is advised just to assure no complicity with this condition. Efforts should be made to reduce triglycerides through the use of omega-3 fatty acids and to normalize vitamin D and magnesium levels.

| NUTRITIONAL SUPPLEMENTS | | |
|---|---|---|
| **Supplement** | **Directions for Use** | **Comments** |
| Vitamin D | 3,000 IU daily | 30-50 ng/mL is normal |
| Chromium picolinate | 400–600 mcg daily. | Lowers the cholesterol level, and improves the HDL/LDL ratio. |
| L-carnitine | 1,000 mg 3 times daily with meals. | Supports cholesterol metabolism, transports essential fatty acids, and aids liver gallbladder function. |
| Lecithin | 1,200 mg 3 times daily before meals. | Emulsifies fat in the body. |
| Niacin | Up to 500 mg daily (before bedtime will reduce the flush feeling) | Raises HDL cholesterol |
| Phosphatide | 1,500 mg daily. | Emulsifies fat in the body. |
| Magnesium | 300 mg daily | helps prevent muscle cramps, improves sleep quality, and supports mental relaxation, reducing stress and anxiety |

| HERBS AND HERBAL SUPPLEMENTS | | |
|---|---|---|
| **Herb** | **Directions for Use** | **Comments** |
| Garlic | Take as directed on the label. | Reduces the cholesterol level. |
| Ginger | Take as directed on the label. | Reduces the cholesterol level. |

## BLEPHARITIS

Blepharitis usually causes symptoms of eye itching, irritation, burning, and a foreign body sensation. Dry eye is also a common complaint and is often worse with contact lens wearers.

The lids may be red and may have ulcerative areas which may actually bleed. Vision is usually normal, although a poor tear film often blurs vision, causing fluctuating vision during the day. Redness, warmth, and swelling in advanced cases may also be noted.

The causes of blepharitis can differ depending on which type of blepharitis is present. Posterior blepharitis is the most common type and usually happens to people who also have Rosacea or another skin disorder. With this version of the condition, the meibomian glands become blocked or secrete a thickened oil that can block the meibomian ducts.

Anterior blepharitis, is caused by the Staphylococcal bacterium. The eyes become infected with this bacterium and a patient will experience a foreign body sensation. This is considered an acute version of the problem and a patient who have a burning sensation in the eyes or matted eyelashes should be prescribed hot compresses, along with a nutrition supplement listed below.

The prevention of blepharitis and treatment of the condition go hand in hand. Regular eye hygiene is the best way to prevent outbreaks of the problem. This should include the chronic blepharitis treatments of daily washing and attention paid to the condition of the lids on a daily basis. For both forms, warm compresses need to be applied to the eyes three to four times a day. With anterior blepharitis, topical antibiotics should be applied to the lid margins for severe infections.

Blepharitis and treatment can also involve some home remedies. One of the most common of these techniques is to use a teabag as the warm compress. The natural astringent factor of the tea will help to liquefy the oils that may be trapped in pores. Chronic blepharitis treatments should be used on a regular basis for anyone who has experienced the symptoms of this condition.

In allergic blepharitis, the lids may appear dark like raccoon eyes, also called an "allergic shiner" and is very common in children. Flaking and "matting" of the lashes are common. In the infectious form, there may be yellow- or green-colored discharge, which causes sticking of the lids, especially in the morning.

With the most common seborrheic form, dry, flaky patches of skin may develop. Blepharitis may localize in the skin of the eyelids causing a stye or a chalazion, which may require incision for drainage. Chronic blepharitis may result in damage of varying severity. This may have a marked negative effect upon the refractive state.

Since blepharitis is essentially a skin condition, nutrients that support healthy skin are in order.

| NUTRITIONAL SUPPLEMENTS | | |
|---|---|---|
| **Supplement** | **Directions for Use** | **Comments** |
| Vitamin A (retinyl palmitate) | 10,000 IU daily | Good for dry skin and epithelial cell integrity |
| Vitamin-B complex | 75 mg daily | Promotes healthy skin and proper circulation. Aids in cellular reproduction |
| Vitamin C with bioflavonoids | 6,000 mg daily in divided doses | An antioxidant; reduces inflammation. *Note:* Use powdered buffered ascorbic acid |
| Copper | 1 mg | Needed to balance zinc (if not monomethionine) |
| Linoleic acid | 500 mg Black Current Seed Oil | Supports skin tissue |
| Omega-3 fish oil | 2,000 mg EPA/DHA daily | Essential fatty acids to support skin cells |
| Zinc (monomethionine) | 40 mg daily. *Caution:* Do not take more than 40 mg daily | Enhances immune function |

| HERBS AND HERBAL SUPPLEMENTS | | |
|---|---|---|
| **Herb** | **Directions for Use** | **Comments** |
| Dulse | Apply as a compress | High in iodine |
| Goldenseal | Apply as a compress | Soothing for the tissues. *Caution:* Do not take internally for more than 1 week. Do not use during pregnancy |
| Horsetail | Apply as a compress | Tones the skin |
| Rosemary | Apply as a compress | Stimulates the skin |
| Sage | Apply as a compress | An astringent |

| HOMEOPATHIC REMEDIES | | |
|---|---|---|
| **Remedy** | **Directions for Use** | **Comments** |
| Antimonium crudum 6c | 3–4 pellets under the tongue 3–4 times daily | Good for all skin conditions |
| Apis mellifica 6c | 3–4 pellets under the tongue 3–4 times daily | Good for all skin conditions |
| Argentum nitricum 6c | 3–4 pellets under the tongue 3–4 times daily | Good for all skin conditions |
| Arsenicum album 6c | 3–4 pellets under the tongue 3–4 times daily | Good for blepharitis associated with anxiety or burning |
| Calcarea sulfurica 6c | 3–4 pellets under the tongue 3–4 times daily | Good for all skin conditions |
| Carboneum sulfuratum 6c | 3–4 pellets under the tongue 3–4 times daily | Good for all skin conditions |
| Euphrasia officinalis 6c | 3–4 pellets under the tongue 3–4 times daily | Good for blepharitis associated with soreness |

| Remedy | Directions for Use | Comments |
|---|---|---|
| Graphites 6c | 3–4 pellets under the tongue 3–4 times daily | Good for all skin conditions |
| Hepar sulphuris 6c | 3–4 pellets under the tongue 3–4 times daily | Good for all skin conditions |
| Lycopodium 6c | 3–4 pellets under the tongue 3–4 times daily | Good for all skin conditions |
| Petroleum 6c | 3–4 pellets under the tongue 3–4 times daily | Good for all skin conditions |
| Rhus toxicodendron 6c | 3–4 pellets under the tongue 3–4 times daily | Good for all skin conditions |
| Sulphur 6c | 3–4 pellets under the tongue 3–4 times daily | Good for all skin conditions |

## RECOMMENDATIONS FOR PATIENTS

- Do not rub your eyes, even if they feel itchy. Severe itching may indicate an allergic reaction.
- Apply a warm compress to your eyes a few times a day, for at least ten minutes each time. To enhance the effect, make a tea of your chosen herb, soak a clean cloth in the tea, and apply the cloth as the compress. When finished, gently wipe the eyelids with the compress to remove any excess debris. Never re-use a compress.
- If itching is the main symptom, use a cold compress.
- Stay away from irritants such as smoke, wind, excessive sunlight, and bright lights.
- Eat a well-balanced diet that emphasizes fresh raw vegetables, plus grains, legumes, and fresh fruits.
- Get sufficient sleep, and avoid eyestrain at least until the severity of the condition improves.

## BLEPHAROSPASM

Blepharospasm is a dystonia caused by abnormal involuntary sustained muscle contractions and spasms. It is both cranial, because it involves the head, and focal, because it is confined to one specific part of the head. Patients with blepharospasm typically have normal eyes; any visual disturbance is solely the repeated forced closure of the eyelids.

Blepharospasm usually begins gradually with excessive blinking and/or eye irritation. In the early stages, it may occur only in the presence of specific stressful conditions, such as bright lights, fatigue, and emotional tension. As the disorder progresses, it occurs more frequently during the day. The spasms disappear during sleep, and some people find that after a good night's slumber, the spasms don't appear for several hours. Concentrating on a specific task often reduces the frequency of the spasms. As the condition progresses further, the spasms may intensify so that when they occur, the patient is functionally blind. The eyelids may even remain forcefully closed for several hours.

### CONVENTIONAL TREATMENT

Botulinum toxin (Botox®) is an approved treatment for blepharospasm in the US and Canada. When it is used to treat blepharospasm, it is injected in minute doses into muscles above and below the eyes. The sites of the injections vary slightly from patient to patient and according to physician preference. The injections are usually given in the eyelid, the brow, and the muscles under the lower lid. The benefits begin one to fourteen days after the treatment and last for an average of three to four months. Long-term follow-up studies have shown the treatment to be very safe and effective, with up to 90 percent of patients obtaining almost complete relief from their blepharospasm.

The side effects of Botox include drooping of the eyelids, blurred vision, and double vision. Excessive tearing may occur. All these side effects are transient, caused mainly by excessive muscle relaxation. Providing the dose is kept small and the injections are given no less than three months apart, this method is effective over a long period of time. The effects of therapy may be increased with the use of some antibiotics or with other drugs that interfere with neuromuscular transmission.

Another treatment option is surgery. However, before considering surgery, it is advisable to try potentially effective non-surgical therapies such as the Botox® injections. Functionally impaired patients with blepharospasm who cannot tolerate or do not respond well to medication or Botox® are candidates for surgical therapy. Current experience has found that this procedure has improved visual disability in 75 to 80 percent of cases of blepharospasm.

## SELF-TREATMENT

One method of self-treatment for blepharospasm is stress reduction. Consider referring the patient out for professional assistance to determine if they have excessive stress in their life. Typical modalities are meditation, breathing techniques, yoga, tai chi, biofeedback, visualization, and counseling. Acupuncture is also a viable alternative to traditional medical treatments.

One study showed that serum calcium levels of the benign essential blepharospasm group were significantly lower than the healthy group. Serum vitamin D levels showed a moderate negative correlation with disease severity. The role of calcium and vitamin D in the evolution of the blepharospasm need further investigation at the cellular and anatomical levels.

| NUTRITIONAL SUPPLEMENTS | | |
|---|---|---|
| **Supplement** | **Directions for Use** | **Comments** |
| Calcium | 1,000 mg daily | For proper muscle function |
| Folic acid | 400 mcg daily | For proper nerve production |
| Magnesium | 250 mg daily | Relaxes muscles |
| Phosphorus | 800 mg daily | For proper nerve growth |
| Potassium | 2,500 mg daily | Rebalances the nerves |
| Vitamin-B complex | 100 mg daily | For stress |

*continued*

| NUTRITIONAL SUPPLEMENTS (*con't*) | | |
|---|---|---|
| **Supplement** | **Directions for Use** | **Comments** |
| Vitamin C with bioflavonoids | 500 mg every 3 hours up to 4 times daily | An antioxidant. *Note:* Use powdered buffered ascorbic acid |
| Vitamin D | 1,000 IU daily | Plays a crucial role in the body's ability to absorb calcium |

| HERBS AND HERBAL SUPPLEMENTS | | |
|---|---|---|
| **Herb** | **Directions for Use** | **Comments** |
| Lobelia | Apply as a compress | Relieves muscle cramping. *Caution:* Do not take internally |
| Valerian | 2-4 grams daily | For relaxation |

| HOMEOPATHIC REMEDIES | | |
|---|---|---|
| **Remedy** | **Directions for Use** | **Comments** |
| Agaricus 6c | 3–4 pellets under the tongue 3–4 times daily. | For eyelid twitching |
| Calcarea carbonica 6c and Magnesia phosphorica 6c | 3–4 pellets of each remedy under the tongue 3–4 times daily. | For blepharospasm associated mineral deficiency |
| Hypericum perforatum 6c | 3–4 pellets under the tongue 3–4 times daily. | For blepharospasm affecting the eye only |
| Ignatia amara 6c | 3–4 pellets under the tongue 3–4 times daily. | For eyelid twitching |
| Nux vomica 6c | 3–4 pellets under the tongue 3–4 times daily. | For eyelid spasm after drinking coffee |
| Physostigma 6c | 3–4 pellets under the tongue 3–4 times daily. | For eyelid twitching |
| Rheum 6c | 3–4 pellets under the tongue 3–4 times daily. | For eyelid twitching |
| Sulphur 6c | 3–4 pellets under the tongue 3–4 times daily. | For eyelid twitching. |

## CATARACTS

Any loss of transparency in the crystalline lens is called a cataract. Cataracts are not limited to the aged, although senile cataract is the most common type of cataract. Between the ages of sixty-five and seventy-four, about 23 percent of the population is expected to have a cataract. After the age of seventy-five, about 50 percent of people will develop a cataract.

Epidemiologic studies of cataract suggest that associated risk factors may include personal characteristics, such as age, sex, race, occupation, and educational status; ocular characteristics, such as iris color, myopic refractive status, diabetes mellitus, hypertension, drug exposure, smoking, and sunlight exposure. Animal and observational epidemiologic studies suggest that deficiencies in vitamins C and E, carotenoids, and the trace elements zinc and selenium also may be associated with the development of cataract. The lens can accumulate minerals such as iron, cadmium calcium and magnesium. This accumulation can eventually lead to cataract formation. Smoking increases iron levels in the lens. Chelation of these minerals may be therapeutic in reversing cataract formation.

If the onset of cataracts could be delayed by 10 years, researchers estimate that half the surgical procedures to remove cataracts could be averted. Cataract surgery is the most common surgical procedure performed in the US. Cataract care costs billions of dollars a year and contribute to hip fractures, auto accidents, and debilitation. Efforts to prevent cataracts are also worthwhile because the eye is a barometer of health and longevity. According to one study, age related cataracts are a marker for increased mortality, up to a 390 percent increase in the death rate. Both AREDS studies included a review of cataract formation as a primary marker. In the cataract portion of the study, researchers discovered that the same nutrients had no significant effect on the development or progression of age-related cataract. This might have been because of the relatively short duration of the study and the fact that the supplements were only taken only once during the day.

Similar to AREDS, the Blue Mountain Eye Study conducted in Australia and published in 2002 featured 3,654 adults 49 years and older examined initially and 2,335 re-examined five years later for nutrient intakes and eye issues. In 2008, using lens photographs taken during these examinations, the research team conducted a specific investigation of cataract incidence and intakes of vitamin, mineral and carotenoid antioxidants. Higher antioxidant intakes had long-term protective associations against development of nuclear cataract, but not incident cortical or posterior subcapsular cataract.

Lutein and zeaxanthin are deposited in the retina as well as in the lens, which might have an impact on cataract risk. These compounds are the only carotenoids detectable in the human lens, although at concentrations considerably lower than in the macula. Their concentration is higher in the cortical lens tissue than in nuclear lens tissue. Clinical findings show that lens optical density is inversely related with MPOD among adults aged 48–72 years. The significance of this association is not yet known but is suggested to be related to processes affecting lens aging.

It has also been shown that estrogen supplementation can reduce the risk of cataract formation. The process might also be related to the modulation of the HDL levels by estrogen in the bloodstream.

Oxidative stress is clearly established as a major factor in cataract development. There have been many studies conducted on nutrition and cataracts. It has been shown, for example, that diets low in vitamin B2 can produce cataracts in animals. In horses, cataracts, which are a common cause of blindness in these animals, can be reduced when large amounts of vitamin B2 are added to the diet. Galactose, a type of milk sugar, increases the need for vitamin B2. In infants who cannot utilize galactose normally, poor vision from cataracts has been corrected by removing milk sugar from the diet and adding vitamin B2.

It has been shown that aqueous humor, the source of nutrition to the lens, contains 26 times more vitamin C than any other bodily fluid. This should be an obvious factor in lens health. In 1991 a study compared 175 cataract patients with 175 age-matched cataract-free individuals.

Researchers found that cataract-free subjects were more likely to be using vitamin C and E supplements. The study suggested at least a 50% reduction in the risk of developing cataracts. In a study reported in 1997, correlating vitamin C intake with cataract formation among 247 women age 56-71 years over a 10-12-year period, only 8% of the women who consumed greater than 359 mg of vitamin C per day obtained their vitamin C solely from food. Most were supplement users. The high-dose supplement users experienced a 77% reduction in cataract risk. Researchers concluded that periods shorter than 10 years are not sufficient to measure the influence of vitamin C upon cataract formation.

Another 1997 study found a significant reduction in cataracts in a group of nurses who took vitamin C supplements. In this study of 478 nurses, age 53 to 73 years, over a period of 13 to 15 years, high vitamin C intake protected against nuclear cataracts. Women using vitamin C supplements for 10 years or more experienced a 64% reduction in their risk to develop nuclear cataracts. High blood plasma levels of ascorbic acid correlated with reduced cataract risk.

Given that human visual system is the most highly valued of the senses, and the lens of the human eye is vulnerable to many oxidative challenges ranging from assault by solar UV radiation, inflammation, elevated blood sugar, ascorbic acid depletion induced by poor diet, and smoking or use of vitamin-depleting drugs (steroids and aspirin are examples), the oral dose of vitamin C to prevent cataracts should be set at the optimal achievable dose to prevent cataracts. It is now apparent that blood concentrations up to or greater than 220 micromole per liter of blood serum can be achieved with serial oral-dose vitamin C. It appears the peak concentration of vitamin C in the aqueous fluid, under static (non- biologically stressed) conditions, is achieved with a 2000 mg oral dose of vitamin C. This dose would need to be repeated throughout the day to achieve an optimal aqueous humor concentration. Possibly 10,000 to 12,000 mg of oral vitamin C would be taken, divided into 2000 mg-doses taken 5 times a day. However, at this dosage, a side effect of diarrhea is likely.

Hickey and Roberts have shown that 500 mg oral dose vitamin C taken 5 times a day, or 2500 mg total, achieves blood plasma levels between 100-140 micromole per liter. This approach appears to be practical and would significantly increase antioxidant protection in the human eye by many times over the suggested 200 mg dietary intake levels. The effect of various adjuvant bioflavonoids such as rutin, found in nature in conjunction with ascorbic acid, also have the potential to prolong the half-life of vitamin C, and must therefore be re-evaluated.

One of the problems with recommendations to supplement with vitamin C to prevent cataracts is that the public is more likely to begin use of supplements after an eye doctor diagnoses cataracts. Cataracts cannot be self-detected. By then, usually in the 6th or 7th decade of life, the hardening, discoloration and opacification of the lens may be irreversible.

Although surgical treatment to remove cataract is very effective, cataract surgery carries risks, such as increased incidence of late-stage macular degeneration. Therefore, many research efforts focus on preventing or slowing cataract development, as well as on determining the causes of cataract formation. It is apparent that, except in those cases of cataracts that are completely congenital, the major factor in the development of the disorder is nutrient imbalance with age.

| NUTRITIONAL SUPPLEMENTS | | |
|---|---|---|
| **Supplement** | **Directions for Use** | **Comments** |
| Alpha-Lipoic Acid | 200 mg daily | Network antioxidant |
| Copper and Manganese | 2 mg of copper and 10 mg of manganese daily | Retard the growth of cataracts |
| Glutathione | As directed on the label | An excellent free-radical scavenger |
| Grape-seed extract | As directed on the label | A powerful antioxidant |
| L-lysine | As directed on the label | Important in collagen formation. Repairs the lens |
| Selenium | 400 mcg daily | A free-radical scavenger |

| Supplement | Directions for Use | Comments |
|---|---|---|
| Superoxide dismutase (SOD) | As directed on the label | A free-radical scavenger. Shown to be very effective at reducing cataract density |
| Magnesium | 500 mg daily | Counteracts excessive calcium deposits |
| N-acetylcarnosine (Can-C) | One drop twice daily | Powerful antioxidant |
| Vitamin A | 3,000 IU daily | Good for all eye conditions |
| Vitamin-B complex with extra B2 | 75 mg of vitamin-B complex B2, and B5 daily | Important for eye metabolism |
| Vitamin C | 5,000 mg 5 times daily | A free-radical scavenger |
| Vitamin E | 400 IU daily | A free-radical scavenger |
| Zinc | 25 mg daily | Protects against light-induced damage. *Caution:* Do not take more than 40 mg daily |

| HERBS AND HERBAL SUPPLEMENTS | | |
|---|---|---|
| **Herb** | **Directions for Use** | **Comments** |
| Bilberry | 100 mg daily | Boosts the circulation. Supplies bioflavonoids, which remove toxic chemicals. *Note:* Use the extract form. |
| Eyebright | Use as an eyewash | Good for overall ocular support |
| Nei zhang ming yan wan (Boiron) | 8 pills 3 times daily | Clarifies the vision. *Caution:* Contains aluminum, so limit its use. |
| Shi hu ye guang wan (Boiron) | 1 pill twice daily | Valuable during the early stages of cataract formation |
| Visioplex Eye Concentrate with Eyebright | 3 pills daily as directed on the label | Promotes the transfer of nutrients to the lens |

| HOMEOPATHIC REMEDIES | | |
|---|---|---|
| **Remedy** | **Directions for Use** | **Comments** |
| Calcarea fluorica 6c | 3–4 pellets under the tongue 3–4 times daily | Supports the connective tissue Restores the integrity of the elastic fibers |
| Calcarea sulfurica 6c | 3–4 pellets under the tongue 3–4 times daily | Supports the connective tissue |
| Causticum 6c | 3–4 pellets under the tongue 3–4 times daily | Good for the elastic fibers |
| Cineraria (Natural Ophthalmics) | 1-2 drops twice daily | Increases circulation, lymph drainage and normal metabolism |
| Magnesia carbonica 6c | 3–4 pellets under the tongue 3–4 times daily | Regulates the acidity of the body fluids |
| Pulsatilla 6c | 3–4 pellets under the tongue 3–4 times daily | Good during the early stages of cataract formation |
| Silicea 6c | 3–4 pellets under the tongue 3–4 times daily | Good for inflammation |
| Sulphur 6c | 3–4 pellets under the tongue 3–4 times daily | Good for cortical cataracts |

## RECOMMENDATIONS FOR PATIENTS

- Avoid dairy products, saturated fats, and any fats or oils that have been subjected to heat, whether during cooking or processing (see below). These foods promote the formation of free radicals, which can damage the lens. Use cold-pressed vegetable oils only.
- The smoke point for some unrefined oils like flaxseed, wheat germ, and walnut oil is low (around 225°F) and many experts say we shouldn't heat them at all. They are rich in polyunsaturated fats and are lovely in smoothies, drizzles, salad dressings, etc.

- Unrefined oils that are higher in monounsaturated fats, like extra virgin olive, are considered medium smoke point oils, which means you can use them for most cooking on the average home stove, including sautéing and pan-frying, slow-roasting in the oven, and even stir-frying as long as you're not cranking the heat over about 375°F.
- Naturally refined oils like coconut, grapeseed, avocado, and sunflower have much higher smoke points, ranging between 400-500°F. Consume 9-13 portions a day of plant-based foods with high antioxidant content. These include: spinach, broccoli, carrots, cantaloupes, and green peppers (all colorful vegetables).
- Avoid antihistamines.
- Avoid steroids for long-term use.
- Diabetics are especially prone to cataracts. Fortunately, pure diabetic cataracts are reversible. Therefore, careful monitoring of the blood-sugar level is critical.
- Avoid sugars--they are pro-inflammatory
- Outdoors on a sunny day, wear a hat with a brim to reduce the dazzle effect of the bright sunlight. Optical quality sunglasses will help with this, too.
- Indoors, have patients experiment with the room lighting. They'll find reading easier if they have a small reading lamp that can be moved around and adjusted for comfort instead of a ceiling fixture that is bright and immovable.

## CENTRAL SEROUS RETINOPATHY

Central serous retinopathy (CSR) involves a collection of fluid under the macula that causes visual distortion. The vision may be minimally to significantly affected, with the visual acuity ranging from 20/20 to 20/200.

CSR affects primarily adults aged twenty to forty-five. Men are affected ten times more frequently than women. Many patients with CSR live under high levels of stress. The exact cause of CSR is controversial. Some experimental evidence suggests that high blood levels of epinephrine and selected hormones may be responsible.

Most CSR patients spontaneously recover their visual acuity within about six months. The average recovery time is three to four months. Many patients have some residual symptoms, such as distortion of shapes and disturbed color vision, contrast sensitivity, and night vision. Despite an overall good prognosis, 40 to 50 percent of patients experience one or more recurrences of the disorder.

No medical therapy has been proven to be effective against CSR. Laser treatment can shorten the duration of the disease, but does not appear to alter the final visual acuity or the recurrence rate. Laser use is controversial because of the potential complications and lack of apparent long-term benefits. Nutritional therapy is designed to support retinal tissue and to reduce swelling.

| NUTRITIONAL SUPPLEMENTS | | |
|---|---|---|
| **Supplement** | **Directions for Use** | **Comments** |
| Longevinex® | 350 mg daily | Good for retinal health |
| Vitamin A | Take 3,000 IU daily | Supports the retina |
| Vitamin-B complex | Take 75 mg daily | Good for stress |
| Vitamin B6 | Take 50–200 mg daily | Reduces fluid retention |
| Vitamin C | Take 2,000–5,000 mg daily | Fortifies the blood vessel walls |
| Vitamin E | Take 200 IU daily | Reduces fluid retention |
| Magnesium | 40 mg daily | Good for stress |
| Zinc | Take 25 mg daily | Good in combination with vitamin A |

| HERBS AND HERBAL SUPPLEMENTS | | |
|---|---|---|
| **Herb** | **Directions for Use** | **Comments** |
| Alfalfa | Drink as a tea | Good for relaxation. Good for chemical imbalance |
| Chamomile | Drink as a tea | Good for relaxation |
| Gotu kola | Drink as a tea | Good for relaxation |
| Lady's slipper | Drink as a tea | Good for relaxation |
| Lobelia | Drink as a tea | Good for relaxation. *Caution*: Do not take internally on an ongoing basis. |
| Passion flower | Drink as a tea | Good for relaxation |
| Valerian | Drink as a tea. | Good for relaxation |

| HOMEOPATHIC REMEDIES | | |
|---|---|---|
| **Remedy** | **Directions for Use** | **Comments** |
| Apis mellifica 6c | 3–4 pellets under the tongue 3–4 times daily | Alleviates swelling |
| Rhus toxicodendron 6c | 3–4 pellets under the tongue 3–4 times daily. | Good for inflammation. Alleviates swelling |
| Sepia 6c | 3–4 pellets under the tongue 3–4 times daily. | Good for inflammation. Alleviates swelling |

## RECOMMENDATIONS FOR PATIENTS

- Use an Amsler Grid to monitor your visual distortion.
- Practice a relaxation technique such as tai chi, yoga, or meditation.
- Practice deep, relaxed breathing.

## CHALAZION

A chalazion results when one of the meibomian gland ducts becomes obstructed. Chalazia are therefore also known as meibomian cysts and should be treated as soon as possible.

Most treatments of a chalazion start with antibiotics, accompanied by hot compresses at least three times a day. Chalazia occasionally grow large enough to obscure vision. At this point, they need to be lanced and drained.

Nutritional support is similar to treating meibomitis: using Omega-3 fish oil in the proper combination with Omega-6 essential fatty acids, along with hot compresses.

| NUTRITIONAL SUPPLEMENTS | | |
|---|---|---|
| **Supplement** | **Directions for use** | **Comments** |
| Omega 3 Essential Fatty Acids | 1500 mg (EPA+DHA) daily | Acts as anti-inflammatory; increases fluidity of meibum |
| Omega-6 (Black Currant Seed Oil) | 350 mg daily | Mucous specific anti-inflammatory |
| Lactoferrin | 40 mg daily | Mucous specific anti-inflammatory |

| HERBS AND HERBAL SUPPLEMENTS | | |
|---|---|---|
| **Herb** | **Directions for Use** | **Comments** |
| Eyebright | Apply as a hot compress | Opens the pores to allow drainage |
| Goldenseal | Apply as a hot compress | Good for eye infections. *Caution:* Do not take internally for more than 1 week. Do not use during pregnancy. |
| Curcumin | 500mg daily | Anti-inflammatory |

| HOMEOPATHIC REMEDIES | | |
|---|---|---|
| **Remedy** | **Directions for Use** | **Comments** |
| Hepar sulphuris 6c | 3–4 pellets under the tongue 3–4 times daily | Good for abscesses, boils, and similar problems |
| Mercurius vivus 6 | 3–4 pellets under the tongue 3–4 times daily | Good for swollen glands, boils, and similar problems |
| Staphysagria 6c | 3–4 pellets under the tongue 3–4 times daily | Good for extremely emotional persons with chalazia |
| Sulphur 6c | 3–4 pellets under the tongue 3–4 times daily | Good for red eyelids |
| Thuja occidentalis 6c | 3–4 pellets under the tongue 3–4 times daily | Good for chalazia associated with warts |

## RECOMMENDATIONS FOR PATIENTS

- Do not rub your eyes with dirty hands, since this can lead to infection.
- Apply a very warm wet washcloth as a compress to the affected eye as soon as possible after first noticing the chalazion. Use a compress often; typically, 3-4 times a day.
- Gently massage the chalazion lump while using a warm compress.
- Check back with the doctor to confirm that the lump is a chalazion.

# COMPUTER VISION SYNDROME

Because computer work visually is such a highly demanding task, vision problems and symptoms are very common. Most studies indicate that computer operators report more eye-related problems than do paper-oriented office workers. A study by the National Institute of Occupational

Safety and Health (NIOSH) showed that 88 percent of computer users complained of computer-related eyestrain. The symptoms generally affecting computer users are now collectively known as Computer Vision Syndrome (CVS), or more recently as Digital Eyestrain (DE). CVS most often occurs when the viewing demand of the task exceeds the visual abilities of the computer user. The AOA defines CVS as that "complex of eye and vision problems related to near work which are experienced during or related to computer use." The symptoms can vary, but usually include eyestrain, headaches, blurred vision (distance and/or near), disturbed accommodation, neck pain and/or backache, light sensitivity, double vision, disturbed color vision, and dry, irritated eyes.

The causes of the inefficiencies and the visual symptoms are a combination of the individuals' visual condition, poor work habits and poor office ergonomics. Many people have marginal vision disorders that do not cause symptoms when performing less demanding visual tasks. In other words, the working environment must be addressed as well as the patient's visual condition when treating CVS.

Since there are many different environmental and visual corrections that can be made to achieve the proper balance for computer use, giving overall recommendations is difficult. However, full time display users have benefited from following a "3-B" approach to reducing eyestrain from computer use. The three 'Bs' are blink, breathe, and break.

- Blink—studies show that display viewers blink about one-third as often as normal. Another study showed that even the blinks that display viewers exhibited were less complete than normal blink closures.
- Breathe—proper breathing can help to relax, not only the eyes, but the whole person. Given the high stress and deadlines of display-based tasks, relaxation is critical.
- Break—studies have shown that shorter, more frequent breaks are more effective than longer, less frequent breaks. The author created the "20-20-20" rule (see below).

It may seem counter-intuitive to think that nutrition may play a role in reducing the incidence or severity of CVS. However, for one example, studies show that a small dose of the carotenoid astaxanthin might have an effect on the visual stress that computer users' exhibit. While astaxanthin is not present within the eye itself, it appears to help with muscular stress, typically in striated muscles. If so, then extra supplementation of astaxanthin might help with extraocular muscle function, therefore. reducing eye fatigue and other CVS symptoms.

Given that blinking is also affected in display viewing, a significant symptom is dry eyes. Some of the recommended nutritional support is for a dry eye condition.

| NUTRITIONAL SUPPLEMENTS | | |
|---|---|---|
| **Supplement** | **Directions for Use** | **Comments** |
| Vitamin A | 3,000 IU daily | Good for conjunctival cell moisture |
| Vitamin-B complex | 75 mg daily | Good for stress |
| Vitamin C | 3,000 mg daily | An antioxidant. Good for stress |
| Vitamin E | 200 IU daily | An antioxidant |
| Astaxanthin | 6 mg daily | Helps maintain muscle tone |
| Capsanthin | 40 mg daily | Relieves dry eyes |

| HERBS AND HERBAL SUPPLEMENTS | | |
|---|---|---|
| **Herb** | **Directions for Use** | **Comments** |
| Eyebright | 3–4 drops daily or apply as a compress | Good for the eye tissues |
| Goldenseal | Apply as a compress | Soothing for the tissues. *Caution:* Do not take internally for more than 1 week. Do not use during pregnancy. |

| HOMEOPATHIC REMEDIES | | |
|---|---|---|
| **Remedy** | **Directions for Use** | **Comments** |
| Euphrasia officinalis 6c | 3–4 pellets under the tongue 3–4 times daily | Alleviates redness |
| Nux vomica 6c | 3–4 pellets under the tongue 3–4 times daily. | Good for eyestrain associated with overwork |
| Ruta graveolens 6c | 3–4 pellets under the tongue 3–4 times daily | Good for eyestrain followed by headache. Heals the tendons and ligaments |
| Sulphur 6c | 3–4 pellets under the tongue 3–4 times daily | Alleviates redness following near-point work |

## RECOMMENDATIONS FOR PATIENTS

- Lower the monitor so that when holding the head in the normal position, the line of sight is just over the top of the monitor.
- The top of the monitor should also be tilted back between 10-15 degrees.
- The viewing distance, in general, should be at least 24 inches away.
- The background illumination of the screen and the illumination of the immediate work area should be approximately equal. They might need to dim the brightness of the screen somewhat, but should also increase the contrast.
- The best screen colors to use are black letters on a white background. This combination simulates paper and ink, and provides the highest contrast between the letters and the background.
- Look for glare on the screen. To check for this, turn the computer off and look for any reflections of lights or lightly colored articles in the screen.

- Address other light hitting your eyes, either directly from a window or lamp, or by reflection off a shiny surface.
- When working at a computer, blink often because this rests and rewets the eyes.
- Breathe fully, since taking complete breaths is important in relaxing the muscles.
- Take breaks from the computer. Use the 20-20-20 rule—every twenty minutes, take twenty seconds and look twenty feet away.

## CONJUNCTIVITIS

Conjunctivitis refers to an inflammation of the conjunctiva that can be caused by a bacterial, viral, or fungal infection; by an allergy; or by anything that has irritated the ocular surface. Most patients will refer to this as "pink eye". It is one of the most common eye infections and is extremely contagious.

The conventional treatment for conjunctivitis generally depends on the source of the condition. Bacterial conjunctivitis is usually treated with antibiotics. Viral conjunctivitis can be treated with antivirals. Fungal forms of conjunctivitis are treated with antifungals. Allergic conjunctivitis is usually treated symptomatically—that is, by reducing the itching and inflammation of the eye along with treating the rest of the allergy symptoms.

The tears contain natural antibacterial enzymes that aid in healing the eye. Nutritional support will vary with the cause of the condition and is designed to support the anterior ocular surface as well as the tear film.

| NUTRITIONAL SUPPLEMENTS | | |
|---|---|---|
| **Supplement** | **Directions for Use** | **Comments** |
| Vitamin A | 3,000 IU daily | Good for epithelial cell support |
| Vitamin C | 2,000–6,000 mg daily in divided doses | Supports tissue healing and the tear film |

(*continued*)

| NUTRITIONAL SUPPLEMENTS (*con't*) | | |
|---|---|---|
| **Supplement** | **Directions for Use** | **Comments** |
| Lactoferrin | 20-40 mg daily | Iron-binding, mucous-specific anti-inflammatory |
| Omega-3 fatty acid | 1000 mg EPA+DHA daily | Supports the tear film |
| Zinc | 25 mg daily | Enhances the immune response |
| Copper | 1 mg daily | Supports zinc use |

| HERBS AND HERBAL SUPPLEMENTS | | |
|---|---|---|
| **Herb** | **Directions for Use** | **Comments** |
| An mian pian (Boiron) | 4 pills 3 times daily | Purges "heat" from the liver |
| Chamomile | Apply as a hot compress or use as an eyewash | Soothing for the eye tissues |
| Eyebright and fennel | Apply as a hot compress or use as an eyewash | Boost the circulation |
| Long dan xie gan wan (Boiron) | 6 pills twice daily | Purges "heat" from the liver and gallbladder |
| Ming mu di huang wan (Boiron) | 10 pills 3 times daily | Good for red or itchy eyes |
| Ming mu shang qing pian (Boiron) | 4 pills twice daily | Good for red, itchy, or burning eyes. *Caution:* Do not use during pregnancy |
| Nei zhang ming yan wan (Boiron) | 8 pills 3 times daily | Good for itchy, painful eyes. *Caution:* Contains aluminum, so limit its use |
| Shi hu ye guang wan (Boiron) | 1 pill twice daily | Good for red or itchy eyes |
| Xiao yao wan (Boiron) | 8 pills 3 times daily | Invigorates a congested liver |

| HOMEOPATHIC REMEDIES | | |
|---|---|---|
| **Remedy** | **Directions for Use** | **Comments** |
| Aconite 6c | 3–4 pellets under the tongue 3–4 times daily. | Good for inflammation |
| Allium cepa 6c | 3–4 pellets under the tongue | Good for inflammation |
| Anacardium 6c | 3–4 pellets under the tongue | Alleviates swelling. |
| Apis mellifica 6c | 3–4 pellets under the tongue | Good for pinkeye with swollen eyelids. Alleviates edema and inflammation |
| Arnica montana 6c | 3–4 pellets under the tongue | Good for inflammation |
| Arsenicum album 6c | 3–4 pellets under the tongue | Good for inflammation |
| Belladonna 6c | 3–4 pellets under the tongue | Good for inflammation |
| Calcarea fluorica 6c | 3–4 pellets under the tongue 3–4 times daily. | Relieves discharge. Good for inflammation |
| Calcarea sulfurica 6c | 3–4 pellets under the tongue 3–4 times daily. | Relieves discharge. Good for inflammation |
| Causticum 6c | 3–4 pellets under the tongue | Relieves discharge |
| Euphrasia officinalis 6c | 3–4 pellets under the tongue 3–4 times daily. | Good for inflammation |
| Graphites 9c | 3-4 pellets under the tongue 3-4 times daily. | Good for inflamed eyelids |
| Mercurius corrosivus 6c | 3–4 pellets under the tongue 3–4 times daily. | Good for pinkeye with mucous discharge. An infection fighter |
| Mercurius vivus 6c | 3–4 pellets under the tongue 3–4 times daily. | Relieves discharge. Good for inflammation |
| Natrum muriaticum 6c | 3–4 pellets under the tongue 3–4 times daily. | Good for inflammation |

(*continued*)

| HOMEOPATHIC REMEDIES (*con't*) | | |
|---|---|---|
| **Remedy** | **Directions for Use** | **Comments** |
| Pulsatilla 6c | 3–4 pellets under the tongue 3–4 times daily. | Relieves discharge. Good for inflammation. Good for allergic conjunctivitis |
| Rhus toxicodendron 6c | 3–4 pellets under the tongue 3–4 times daily. | Good for inflammation. Alleviates swelling |
| Ruta graveolens 6c | 3–4 pellets under the tongue 3–4 times daily. | Good for inflammation |
| Sepia 6c | 3–4 pellets under the tongue 3–4 times daily. | Good for inflammation. Alleviates swelling |
| Silicea 6c | 3–4 pellets under the tongue 3–4 times daily. | Good for inflammation |
| Sulphur 6c | 3–4 pellets under the tongue 3–4 times daily. | Good for inflammation. Good for allergic conjunctivitis |

## RECOMMENDATIONS FOR PATIENTS

- Conjunctivitis is one of the most contagious diseases currently known. Children seem to be more susceptible to it, probably due to their lack of proper hygiene. Children should be counseled to wash their hands properly and to keep the hands away from the eyes.
- For allergic reactions, cold-water rinses can be very effective (following good hand scrubbing). However, counsel patients to NOT use an "eyecup" because it will harbor the allergen and may cause the problem to recur.

- If itching is a symptom, be sure to counsel patients to clean their hands and face often, and splash their eyes with cold water. *Do not* recommend using any over-the-counter preparations that promise to remove "redness" from the eyes. Discourage using Lumify until the infection is controlled.
- Patients can try to treat conjunctivitis with a hot compress two or three times a day. Suggest this treatment specifically if their lids are sticking together in the morning. However, if the condition doesn't resolve within a few days, stronger treatment is indicated.

## CORNEAL ABRASION

A corneal abrasion is any disruption on the cornea surface. Patients often complain that something is "under the upper eyelid". Oftentimes, the foreign body is no longer present but the patient feels some discomfort when the eyelid passes over the abraded area.

Most corneal abrasions heal within a day or two, although injuries from a plant material such as wood or a very dirty substance may take longer. If needed, some form of NSAID or another OTC anti-inflammatory will calm the patient. Nutritional support is directed toward healing the wound and strengthening the corneal tissue.

| NUTRITIONAL SUPPLEMENTS | | |
|---|---|---|
| **Supplement** | **Directions for Use** | **Comments** |
| Vitamin A drops (retinoic acid) | 1–2 drops 3–4 times daily for 2 days | Supports the corneal tissue as it heals |
| Vitamin C | 500 mg twice daily for 2 days | Builds collagen tissue |
| Vitamin B2 | 75 mg daily | Helps collagen crosslinking |
| Omega-3 essential fatty acids | 1000 mg (EPA+DHA) daily | Supports the tear film |
| Lactoferrin | 20 mg oral | Mucous tissue anti-inflammatory |

| HERBS AND HERBAL SUPPLEMENTS | | |
|---|---|---|
| **Herb** | **Directions for Use** | **Comments** |
| Bayberry, eyebright, and goldenseal | Use as an eyewash twice daily | Good for all eye conditions. *Caution:* Do not take goldenseal internally for more than 1 week. Do not use goldenseal during pregnancy. |
| Comfrey | Use as an eyewash | Promotes healing |
| White willow bark | 400 mg as needed | Good for pain |

| HOMEOPATHIC REMEDIES | | |
|---|---|---|
| **Remedy** | **Directions for Use** | **Comments** |
| Aconite 6c | 3–4 pellets under the tongue 3–4 times daily | Good for general eye discomfort |
| Aurum 6c | 3–4 pellets under the tongue 3–4 times daily | Good for pain |
| Belladonna 6c | 3–4 pellets under the tongue 3–4 times daily | Good for pain |
| Bryonia 6c | 3–4 pellets under the tongue 3–4 times daily | Good for pain |
| Chamomilla 6c | 3–4 pellets under the tongue 3–4 times daily | Good for pain |
| Cinchona officinalis 6c | 3–4 pellets under the tongue 3–4 times daily | Good for pain |
| Hypericum perforatum 6c | 3–4 pellets under the tongue 3–4 times daily | Good for nerve injury |
| Lycopodium 6c | 3–4 pellets under the tongue 3–4 times daily | Good for pain |
| Mercurius vivus 6c | 3–4 pellets under the tongue 3–4 times daily | Good for corneal abrasions accompanied by discharge |
| Natrum muriaticum 6c | 3–4 pellets under the tongue 3–4 times daily | Good for pain |

| Remedy | Directions for Use | Comments |
|---|---|---|
| Nitricum acidum 6c | 3–4 pellets under the tongue 3–4 times daily | Good for pain |
| Sanguinaria 6c | 3–4 pellets under the tongue 3–4 times daily | Good for pain. |
| Staphysagria 6c | 3–4 pellets under the tongue3–4 times daily | Good for corneal abrasions associated with anger. |
| Spigelia 6c | 3–4 pellets under the tongue 3–4 times daily | Good for pain. |

## RECOMMENDATIONS FOR PATIENTS

- Get plenty of rest, including a good night's sleep.
- Take an over-the-counter pain medication if the homeopathic remedies aren't effective enough or if your eye is still very uncomfortable.
- Use a cool compress to calm the eye and to reduce the inflammation.
- If your eye doesn't feel "normal" again in twenty-four to thirty-six hours, return to the clinic.

## CORNEAL NEOVASCULARIZATION

Even a slight amount of blood vessel growth into the edges of the cornea indicates that the amount of oxygen reaching the cornea has decreased. This most commonly occurs with contact lens over-wear. A small amount of growth is not normally considered significant or a threat to vision. However, if left unchecked, the growth could continue until blood vessels have grown throughout the cornea.

The main goal of nutritional support of the cornea is increasing the oxygen supply to the cornea. Obviously, contact lens wear should cease until the corneal oxygenation is re-established. Switching to a daily disposable modality should be considered a priority.

| NUTRITIONAL SUPPLEMENTS | | |
|---|---|---|
| **Supplement** | **Directions for Use** | **Comments** |
| Vitamin A | Take 3,000 IU daily | Supports epithelial cell integrity |
| Vitamin C | 3,000 mg daily in divided doses | Maintains collagen stability |
| Vitamin E | 200 IU daily | Fortifies the blood vessel walls |
| Omega-3 fatty acid | 1000-2000 mg daily | Supports the tear film |

| HERBS AND HERBAL SUPPLEMENTS | | |
|---|---|---|
| **Herb** | **Directions for Use** | **Comments** |
| Eyebright | Use as an eyewash. | Good for all eye conditions. |

| HOMEOPATHIC REMEDIES | | |
|---|---|---|
| **Remedy** | **Directions for Use** | **Comments** |
| Aconite 6c | 3–4 pellets under the tongue 3–4 times daily | Alleviates redness. |
| Apis mellifica 6c | 3–4 pellets under the tongue 3–4 times daily | Alleviates swelling. |

## RECOMMENDATIONS FOR PATIENTS

- Don't wait until your contact lenses start to irritate your eyes before getting them evaluated.
- Check with your doctor at the first sign of redness or discomfort in your eyes.

## CORNEAL ULCER

The most common cause of corneal ulcers today is related to contact lens wearing. The lens being in constant contact with the corneal surface, combined with poor lens hygiene and/or extended wearing time, can lead to a break in the corneal surface.

Corneal ulcers require a rapid response with proper medical treatment. In conjunction with urgent intervention, nutritional support is important in the healing process. Don't forget to have patients consider lifestyle changes to aid in resolving the condition.

| NUTRITIONAL SUPPLEMENTS | | |
|---|---|---|
| **Supplement** | **Directions for Use** | **Comments** |
| Folic acid | 5 mg 3 times daily | Aids tissue healing |
| Vitamin A | 3,000 IU daily | Good for all eye conditions |
| Vitamin B2 | 100 mg daily | Aids nerve healing and corneal structure |
| Vitamin C | 4,000 mg divided doses through day | Aids tissue healing |
| Vitamin E | 400 IU daily | Aids tissue healing |
| Omega-3 essential fatty acids | 1,000-3,000 mg (EPA+DHA) daily | Anti-inflammatory; supports the anterior ocular surface |

| HERBS AND HERBAL SUPPLEMENTS | | |
|---|---|---|
| **Herb** | **Directions for Use** | **Comments** |
| Eyebright | 1–2 drops 4–5 times daily | Good for overall eye healing. *Note:* Begin taking after you have finished taking other drops |

| HOMEOPATHIC REMEDIES | | |
|---|---|---|
| **Remedy** | **Directions for Use** | **Comments** |
| Aconite 6c | 3–4 pellets under the tongue 3–4 times daily | Alleviates pain and inflammation in the early stages of corneal-ulcer formation |
| Apis mellifica 6c | 3–4 pellets under the tongue 3–4 times daily | Good for inflammation |
| Calcarea sulfurica 6c | 3–4 pellets under the tongue 3–4 times daily | Reduces light sensitivity |
| Euphrasia officinalis 6c | 3–4 pellets under the tongue 3–4 times daily | Good for all eye conditions |
| Mercurius corrosivus 6c | 3–4 pellets under the tongue 3–4 times daily | Good for pain |

## RECOMMENDATIONS FOR PATIENTS

- If you experience any sharp pain and discomfort around the eyes, return to the clinic immediately.
- If you wear contact lenses and feel discomfort, remove the lenses immediately and don't reinsert them until your eyes feel comfortable again. If your eyes continue to feel uncomfortable, see your doctor.
- The best thing you can do if you have a corneal ulcer is to follow your doctor's advice exactly. Ulcers can cause permanent vision loss if they are not dealt with quickly and effectively, so pay attention to all of your doctor's instructions.
- Keep excessive makeup away from the eye area, and be sure not to touch the eye area with unwashed fingers. Once the main episode has resolved and the healing process has begun, you can use some supplemental support to speed up the healing.

## DIABETIC RETINOPATHY

The global prevalence of diabetes has been increasing and is projected to rise to 366 million people by 2030, a 39% increase since 2000. Unless this trend is reversed, the number of people afflicted with diabetic retinopathy is likely to climb as well. It has been shown that 26% of diabetics have diabetic retinopathy. Diabetic retinopathy is the leading cause of blindness in working-age adults.

Laser therapy (PRP) has been the primary means of treating diabetic retinopathy and can reduce the progression of the condition to the more serious proliferative form and blindness. Without treatment, however, the condition only worsens. A long-term epidemiological study in the US found an 86% rate of progression of diabetic retinopathy over 14 years of follow-up.

In theory, antioxidants might be beneficial in this condition by retarding oxidative damage to the retinal vasculature. A cross-sectional study that evaluated plasma carotenoids in 111 individuals with type 2 diabetes found that levels of xanthophyll carotenoids (like lutein and zeaxanthin) were significantly lower in the retinopathy group than carotene carotenoids (alpha-carotene, beta-carotene, lycopene and beta-cryptoxanthin). In addition, a higher xanthophyll carotenoid to carotene carotenoids ratio predicted a lower risk of diabetic retinopathy and vice versa. The authors suggested that synergies among antioxidants, carotenoids are implicated in diabetic retinopathy, independent of other factors.

No significant association was identified between serum vitamin C levels and diabetic retinopathy in two epidemiological studies; nor are there any relevant clinical studies of antioxidants and diabetic retinopathy, according to a Cochrane review.

Some studies have suggested a link between the microvascular damage characteristic of retinopathy and elevated homocysteine levels in the blood. Two studies found an association between elevated homocysteine in the more severe forms of the disease proliferative retinopathy and proliferative retinopathy with macular edema. However, neither one found any association with lipoic acid, vitamin B6 more vitamin B12, the vitamins involved in homocysteine metabolism.

In general, reducing the overall physical effects of diabetes will consequently alter the retinal ramifications of the disease process. It is well documented that body mass index (BMI) and obesity in general contribute to the incidence of diabetes, and the retinal degenerative changes occur increasingly with the length of disease process. If treated properly with alternations of lifestyle factors of smoking, high carbohydrate intake, decreased exercise, etc. the process of the disease can actually reverse, and possibly save the vision of the individual.

Early in diabetes, before the blood sugar is brought under control, diabetics often experience blurred vision. This is because the high blood sugar causes fluid retention changes in the crystalline lens. Blurred vision may, in fact, be the first sign of diabetes. After the proper insulin dosage is determined and the disease is stabilized, the blurred visual changes resolve, although it may recur if the blood sugar rises again.

Diabetic retinopathy typically occurs about ten to twelve years into the disorder but sometimes sooner. If left unchecked, retinal hemorrhages and fluid leaks will eventually spill into the vitreous where they can scar and often cause retinal detachment and blindness.

The best treatment for diabetes is to prevent it from beginning in the first place. There is evidence that staying in good diabetic control—that is, keeping the blood-sugar level normal through diet and insulin—minimizes the long-term, as well as short-term, complications of the disorder. There is also a slight hereditary factor, so if your patient has a parent with diabetes, they are automatically at high risk and should be especially careful to eat a healthy diet and get regular medical checkups. However, environmental factors tend to play more of a role in the development of diabetes than do genetic factors.

More about diabetes can be found in the Diets chapter: "Nutrition for the Diabetic Patient"

| Nutritional Supplements | | |
|---|---|---|
| **Supplement** | **Directions for Use** | **Comments** |
| Alpha-Lipoic Acid | 200 mg daily | Improves blood sugar control |
| Chromium picolinate | 400-600 mcg daily | Improves insulin efficiency |
| Longevinex® | 350 mg daily | Supports retinal structures |
| Magnesium | 500 mg daily | Protects against arterial spasm |
| Manganese | 4 mg daily | An enzyme activator |
| Niacin | 20 mg daily | Small amounts increase circulation |
| Potassium | 300 mg daily | Maintains proper fluid balance |
| Selenium | 100 mcg daily | Suppresses development of new blood vessels |
| Vitamin A | 3,000 IU daily | Recommended for diabetics, who often have difficulty converting beta-carotene to vitamin A |
| Vitamin B-complex | 75 mg daily | Boosts circulation |
| Vitamin D | 5,000 IU daily | Necessary for proper blood clotting. |
| Vitamin E | 400 IU daily | Antioxidant; Aids tissue healing |

| Herbs and Herbal Supplements | | |
|---|---|---|
| **Herb** | **Directions for Use** | **Comments** |
| Cinnamon | Up to 6 grams daily | Improves glucose and lipids in diabetes patients |
| Comfrey | Drink as a tea | Strengthens the blood |
| Dandelion | Drink as a tea | Boosts the activity of the pancreas. |
| Ginseng | Drink as a tea | Normalizes the blood. |
| Gymnema sylvestre | Drink as a tea | Helps the pancreas produce insulin |
| Yarrow | Drink as a tea | Controls bleeding. |

| HOMEOPATHIC REMEDIES | | |
|---|---|---|
| **Remedy** | **Directions for Use** | **Comments** |
| Lachesis 6c | 3-4 pellets under the tongue 3-4 times daily. | Restores vascular integrity. |
| Natrum sulfuricum 6c | 3-4 pellets under the tongue 3-4 times daily. | Supports pancreatic function. |
| Phosphorus 6c | 3-4 pellets under the tongue 3-4 times daily. | Improves metabolism of the vascular tissue. |
| Syzygium jambolanum 6c | 3-4 pellets under the tongue 3-4 times daily. | Supports sugar metabolism |
| Uranium nitricum 6c | 3-4 pellets under the tongue 3-4 times daily. | Acts as a glucose stabilizer. |

## RECOMMENDATIONS FOR PATIENTS

- Since diabetes is a systemic disease, even the control of diabetic eye changes is initially done using general treatments such as diet and exercise.
- Consult with a nutritionist who has a program specifically for managing diabetes.
- Have your blood sugar level checked regularly, especially if diabetes runs in your family.
- If you notice any fluctuations in your vision, either day-to-day or within the day, request that you be tested for diabetes.
- Once you are diagnosed with diabetic retinopathy, you should have a dilated eye exam once a year, and more often if recommended by your doctor.

# DIGITAL EYESTRAIN

*See* Computer Vision Syndrome

## DRY EYE DISEASE

Dry eye disease (DED) is a problem with either the quantity or quality of the tear film, leading to the symptoms of dryness, redness, burning, grittiness, and excessive tearing. At one time, dry eye "syndrome" was not considered so much a disease, but a group of symptoms that develops as a result of another condition such as an allergy or arthritis, the use of medication, or environmental factors such as low humidity or computer use. We now know that it can be a specific disease process (with inflammation) and can be exaggerated by these conditions.

It is important to distinguish between dry eye disease and dry eye syndrome. There are differences between the two conditions, as noted in the chart below:

| **Dry Eye Disease** | **Dry Eye Syndrome** |
|---|---|
| Occurs daily | Mostly during the work week |
| Associated with inflammatory markers | No inflammatory markers |
| Lubrication ineffective | Lubrication effective for a short time |
| Any environment | Specific environments |
| Not computer-use related | Worse with computer use |
| Can be related to prescription medications | No prescriptions taken |

Traditionally, dry eye treatment required treatment in the form of artificial tears or pharmaceutical solutions used to restore tear production and comfort. Anything other than this was contrary to belief and intuition.

As science has revealed more about the genesis of degenerative diseases, however, we have realized that the ocular and periorbital glands respond to stress and degenerative change. Age, stress, and degeneration appear to be related to a build-up of free radicals in tissue at the cellular level. This results in loss of function and premature aging of tissues. Chronic DED may be the result of such changes. Other stress-producing factors may be corneal surgery and contact lens wear.

Scientific studies indicate that one of the major contributors to the accumulation of free radicals in the lacrimal, mucous and oil-producing glands of the eye and orbit may be nutritional deficiency. Scientific research over the past several decades has shown that specifically targeted nutritional supplements can restore function to the glands providing lubrication to the eye. It is this research that has led to the identification of specific nutrient antioxidants that can restore and support improved tear function.

In treating dry eyes, it is important to consider the entire anterior ocular system, not just replacement of tears alone. The chronic inflammatory component of dry eye has only recently been addressed.

## ESSENTIAL FATTY ACIDS

Oral nutritional formulations of Essential Fatty Acids (EFAs) are being used to treat dry eye syndrome—some with more success than others. EFAs as an effective treatment for dry eye disease is dependent on the proper balance of both Omega 6 and Omega 3 EFAs from chemically stable plant oil to consistently produce Series One tear-specific anti-inflammatory prostaglandin (PGE 1). EFA formulations will also block Arachidonic Acid (AA) fatty acid cleavage to the Series Two Cyclooxygenase enzyme (COX2), which can convert to a pro-inflammatory Series Two prostaglandin (PGE 2) without the nutrient co-factors that inhibit the formation of COX 2. (See the chart below to refresh your understanding of the metabolism of EFAs in the treatment of dry eyes.)

In addition to EFAs, nutrient co-factors also stimulate the production of healthy goblet cells, as well as enhance production of clearer and thinner meibomian gland oil production. Properly designed formulations will also stimulate lacrimal gland secretion, as well as stimulate the production of tear lactoferrin, the anti-viral, anti-bacterial iron-binding protein that is particularly vital to the LASIK and other post-operative patients. Abnormal levels of lactoferrin in the body are related to some serious diseases, such as inflammatory bowel disease, Alzheimer's disease and dry eye disease. Recent studies indicate that lactoferrin can be used as a biomarker for diagnosis of these diseases. Dry eye nutritional formulations that are based on the most recent science now include iron-free lactoferrin in the product. Serum lactoferrin is released from the eyelid in a manner similar to serum IgG, and possibly from tear neutrophils during infection and inflammation, and by binding iron, prevents the pathogen from obtaining sufficient iron for growth.

The nutritional formulations that are designed around chemically stable Omega 6 plant oils all contain Linoleic Acid (LA) and significant amounts of Gamma Linolenic Acid (GLA), plus the nutrient co-factors necessary to ensure the Delta 6 Desaturase (D6D) enzymatic metabolic conversion to the tear specific anti-inflammatory PGE 1. They also contain varying amounts of Omega 3 Alpha Linolenic Acid (ALA), which converts to Docosahexaenoic Acid (DHA) and Eicosapentaenoic Acid (EPA). To back up this plant-based ALA/DHA/EPA conversion, formulations should include small amounts of mercury-free fish oil, which contains DHA and EPA, necessary to block the Delta-5-Desaturase (D5D) enzymatic AA cleavage of the Omega 6 downstream Dihomo-Gamma-Linolenic Acid (DGLA) metabolite by the COX 2 enzyme. This enzyme, if not blocked, can convert both Omega 6 DGLA and Omega 3 Stearidonic Acid EFA to the pro-inflammatory series two prostaglandins (PGE 2). Many dry eye nutritional products do not address the AA/COX 2 cleavage issues as they pertain to the downstream conversion of EFA to anti-inflammatory prostaglandins.

Some formulations are focused on the metabolic action of the Omega 3s primarily found in flax and fish oils. The Omega 3 also requires nutrient co-factors to consistently convert downstream to DHA and EPA, which subsequently convert to the anti-inflammatory series three prostaglandins (PGE 3). PGE 3 is an important site-specific anti-inflammatory, particularly for the rheumatoid arthritis patient, but not as specific to tears as the series one prostaglandins from the Omega 6 fatty acid metabolites.

Some practitioners are still using flax oil as a stand-alone treatment for dry eye syndrome because it contains a large amount of Omega 3 and a small amount of Omega 6. Unfortunately, flax oil is highly unstable and contains none of the nutrient co-factors necessary to ensure the consistent enzymatic conversion to either the series one (PGE 1) or the series three (PGE 3) anti-inflammatory prostaglandin, nor does it enhance the production of tear lactoferrin. The same can be said for any of the plant-based Omega 3 fatty acids.

## SEA BUCKTHORN

Palmitoleic acid (POA, 16:1 n-7) is a beneficial monounsaturated fatty acid that acts as part of the body's "rescue system" to improve metabolic health. It enhances insulin sensitivity, reduces inflammation, and helps manage fatty liver disease. It is found in macadamia nuts, dairy, and sea buckthorn oil. Recent studies have shown that oral intake of sea buckthorn pulp oil (not seed oil) restored aqueous tear secretion to its normal value under dry eye conditions. Those results suggest that sea buckthorn pulp oil has a potency to preserve tear secretion levels in dry eye.

The results of studies on Sea Buckthorn oil indicate that the positive effects on dry eye are not mediated through direct effects on the tear film fatty acids. Carotenoids and tocopherols in the oil or eicosanoids produced from the fatty acids of the oil may have a positive effect on inflammation and differentiation of the meibomian gland cells.

## VITAMIN D

It might also be considered efficacious to evaluate a dry eye patient for vitamin D levels. Studies have shown a correlation with low vitamin D levels and dry eye symptoms. After oral intake, vitamin D is rapidly and well absorbed in the small intestine, with plasma levels peaking around 24 h after administration. It is suggested to take vitamin D with fatty foods to enhance absorption.

| NUTRITIONAL SUPPLEMENTS | | |
|---|---|---|
| **Supplement** | **Directions for Use** | **Comments** |
| Omega-3 | 2-3,000 mg daily | High in essential fatty acids. Increases lipid layer |
| Capsanthin | 40 mg daily | Shown to enhance lipid layer |
| Coenzyme Q10 | 80 mg daily | A powerful antioxidant |
| Black Current Seed Oil | 1,000 mg daily at bedtime | Supplies essential fatty acids |
| Iodine | 75 mcg per day | Tear glands contain iodine |
| Sea Buckthorn Oil | 400 mg daily | Supports meibomian glands |
| Vitamin A | 3,000 IU | Supports corneal epithelial cells |
| Vitamin B6 | 50 mg daily | Regulates kidney function |
| Vitamin C | 7,500 mg daily-evenly divided throughout the day | An antioxidant |
| Vitamin D | 400-600 IU daily | modulates immune and inflammatory responses |

| HERBS AND HERBAL SUPPLEMENTS | | |
|---|---|---|
| **Herb** | **Directions for Use** | **Comments** |
| Chamomile | Use warm as an infusion or cool as an eyewash. | Supports the eye tissues |
| Goldenseal | Use warm as an infusion or cool as an eyewash. | Supports the eye tissues. *Caution:* Do not take internally for more than 1 week. Do not use during pregnancy |
| Ming mu di huang wan (Boiron) | 10 pills 3 times daily or drink as a tea. | Builds "yin" in the kidneys, and "cools" the liver |
| Qi ju di huang wan (Boiron) | 8 pills 3 times daily or drink as a tea. | Builds "yin" in the kidneys, and "cools" the liver |
| Shi hu ye guang wan (Boiron) | 1 pill twice daily | Good for all eye conditions |

| HOMEOPATHIC REMEDIES | | |
|---|---|---|
| **Remedy** | **Directions for Use** | **Comments** |
| Aconite 6c | 3–4 pellets under the tongue 3–4 times daily | Alleviates dryness |
| Alumina 6c | 3–4 pellets under the tongue 3–4 times daily | Alleviates dryness |
| Arsenicum album 6c | 3–4 pellets under the tongue 3–4 times daily | Alleviates dryness |
| Belladonna 6c | 3–4 pellets under the tongue 3–4 times daily | Good for dry eyes associated with fever and redness |
| Dry Eye Formula (Natural Ophthalmics) | 1-2 drops daily as needed for relief | Two different formulas: for men and for women |
| Euphrasia officinalis 6c | 3–4 pellets under the tongue 3–4 times daily | Good for dry eyes associated with wind (gas) |
| Optique 1 (Boiron) | 1–2 drops daily as needed for relief | A good general remedy |
| Pulsatilla 6c | 3–4 pellets under the tongue 3–4 times daily | Alleviates dryness |
| Similisan No. 1 | 1–2 drops daily as needed for relief | Good for red, dry eyes |
| Sulphur 6c | 3–4 pellets under the tongue 3–4 times daily | Alleviates dryness, and reduces redness |
| Veratrum album 6c | 3–4 pellets under the tongue 3–4 times daily | Alleviates dryness |
| Zincum metallicum 6c | 3–4 pellets under the tongue 3–4 times daily | Alleviates dryness |

## RECOMMENDATIONS FOR PATIENTS

- Use preservative-free eye drops for lubrication.
- If you have dry eyes, contact your eye doctor before changing your diet. In addition to your specific eye condition, your medical history, prescription medications, and allergies all need to be taken into account.
- Use humidifiers in your home. This is especially important if you live in a dry area or at high altitudes.
- Wear wraparound sun goggles outdoors. Sunglasses (or even clear goggles) with side shields can help reduce the evaporation of moisture from the eye by as much as 40%.
- Blink! When you blink, you squeeze out tears from the glands in your eyelids. Waiting twenty to thirty seconds between blinks may cause the tear film to break, which can lead to dehydration of the surface of the eye.
- Quit smoking. Cigarette smoke causes dry spots to develop on the surface of the eye 40-percent faster than when the lids are held open.
- Avoid smog and fumes. Smog and fumes not only cause dry and irritated eyes; they also inactivate the enzyme that acts as an antibacterial agent in the tear fluid.
- Check the nose pads on your eyeglasses. If your lower eyelids are pushed down by the nose pads of your glasses, you may experience increased evaporation of tears. Have an optician adjust the pads.
- Reposition your computer monitor. If you use a desktop computer, position the monitor so that your eyes aim downward when you look at the center of the screen. This will allow you to keep your eyes partially closed, reducing the surface area of the eye exposed to the air.

- Reduce, replace, or avoid eye makeup. Eye makeup has been shown to thin out the oily layer of the tear film, the outer layer that keeps the eyes from becoming dehydrated. It can harbor bacteria and should be replaced frequently. Gentle removal of all eye makeup every night is essential.
- Check your medications. Some medications can cause dry eyes as a side effect. These medications include antihistamines; atropine; beta blockers; cancer medications; codeine; decongestant eye drops; decongestants; morphine; allergy medications; scopolamine; tranquilizers; and vitamin A analogs. The artificial sweetener aspartame, excessive supplemental vitamin B3, and the cannabis intake can also cause dry eyes.
- Check your soft contact lenses. Soft contact lenses often promote the evaporation of tears from the surface of the eye. In severe dry eye cases, contact lenses cannot be worn. Ask your doctor to recommend a lens that is indicated for dry eyes.
- Check your diet. Avoid consuming margarine, fried foods, and saturated fats in general. The body requires the consumption of essential oils for lubrication of the joints and the eyes, and for restoration of normal lubrication to the body. There are good fats and bad fats. The undesired fats, called saturated fats, are found in some meats, fried foods, butter, dairy products, and margarine. The good fats, especially the omega 3 oils, are polyunsaturated and are found in cold-water fish, ground flaxseeds, and walnuts. There has been a large amount of debate on the nutritional aspects of treating dry eyes but we now know that the fish oils and seed-oil based Omega 6 essential fatty acids, in the right combination can effectively treat this condition.

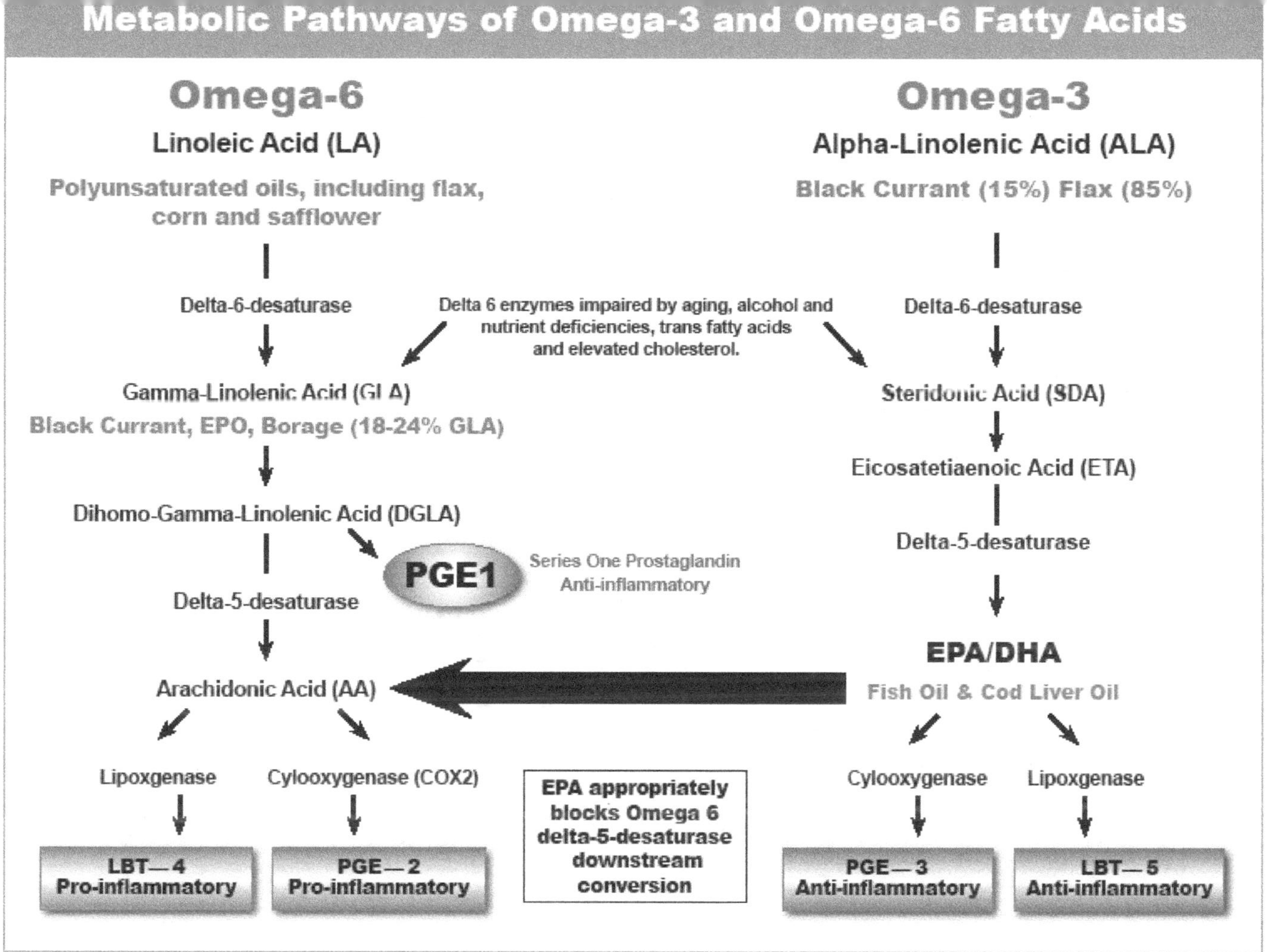


**Figure 1.** Metabolic Pathways of Omega-3 and Omega-6 Fatty Acids. COURTESY BIOSYNTRX, INC.

## FLOATERS

Patients often talk about seeing small dark spots in front of their eyes that seem to move as their eyes move. These spots may be described as dots, squiggles, strands, or any of hundreds of other different shapes, and they are very common. Patients just need to be aware of how these visual effects are determined.

Floaters can also occur when protein fibers from the gel in the vitreous clump together. Floaters may be more obvious when viewing bright areas, such as a blank wall or the white pages of a book, and they may even be seen when the eyes are closed, especially in a bright light or lying in the sun. This happens when these strands float closer to the retina and toward the macula.

Although floaters do not normally increase in number with age, oftentimes they seem to become more apparent. The reason for this is that the vitreous of the eye liquifies with age. This allows the floaters to move more freely and to more frequently get into the line of sight.

If a patient presents with a chief complaint of floaters, a full dilated fundus exam is indicted. The differential diagnosis is retinal detachment and vitreous detachment.

### CONVENTIONAL TREATMENT

A 2019 study from Taiwan suggested that eating pineapple may help reduce eye floaters. The study found that participants who ate pineapple daily for three months experienced a 55–70% reduction in floaters. The rationale here is that because the pineapple contains an enzyme called bromelain. The bromelain can digest proteins, specifically collagen, and eye floaters are made of collagen. Thus, the researchers thought, maybe eating pineapple chunks daily would allow the bromelain to digest the floaters. However, more studies are needed to confirm these findings. Other nutrients include vitamin C, beta-carotene, and vitamin A, which may reduce the risk of vision loss. However, there is no scientific validation that the bromelain in eating pineapple will make its way into the vitreous.

One study looked at various antioxidants and amino acids to reduce floaters. The results were "weak" but some people noted a positive subjective response. Some of those nutrients are listed in the chart below.

A diet rich in fruits and vegetables may help prevent, reduce, or eliminate eye floaters. Floaters are harmless, and there is no practical treatment for them. One word of caution, however—if patients complain of *a lot* of floaters that appear all of a sudden or are associated with flashes of light in their vision, a dilated exam and/or ER visit is warranted.

Within the past several years a specific laser therapy has been promoted. The technique uses a Nd-YAG laser in the process called vitreolysis. The Scanning Laser Ophthalmoscope (SLO) is used to locate the position, the size and the motility of the vitreous floaters with respect to the patient's visual axis. With this technique it is possible to define more precisely some eligibility criteria for Nd-YAG laser treatment of vitreous floaters and to classify the vitreous floaters in ill-suspended and well-suspended floaters in the vitreous body. The well-suspended floaters responding better to treatment compared to the ill-suspended vitreous floaters. While it can be used to benefit some patients, it is still a high-risk procedure and not all floaters can be addressed with this technique. Consultation with a non-participating surgeon is recommended.

## NUTRITIONAL SUPPLEMENTS

The vitreous consists mostly of collagen. The body naturally synthesizes collagen protein by combining the amino acids proline and glycine. Therefore, ensuring adequate intake of these amino acids will support endogenous collagen production. While there are plant-based sources of proline such as wheat germ and some vegetables like asparagus, the proline content is much higher in egg whites and dairy products. Glycine is particularly high in animal skin (chicken skin, pork skin) and gelatin. However, it is also present in most protein-rich foods. Vegans and vegetarians may be able to meet the needs of these amino acids through diet, but if not, collagen supplements can help.

Here is a list of nutrients that help with collagen structure: Calcium, Magnesium, Boron, Silica, Chromium, Potassium, Selenium, Vitamin C, Bioflavonoids, Manganese, Vitamin D, Zinc, Copper, and Vitamin E

| NUTRITIONAL SUPPLEMENTS | | |
|---|---|---|
| **Nutrient** | **Dosage** | **Comments** |
| Vitamin C | 40 mg daily | Antioxidant |
| Grape Seed Extract | 26 mg | Reduces glycation |
| Hesperidin | 100 mg | Antioxidant |
| L-lysine | 125 mg daily | Essential amino acid |
| Zinc | 5 mg | Antioxidant and antiglycation properties |

## RECOMMENDATIONS TO PATIENTS

- When a patient becomes aware of floaters in their field of vision, have them try to just quickly look away, and then back at what they were viewing. This is often enough to move the floaters out of the way—until they float back into the field of vision once again!

# GLAUCOMA

Glaucoma is an umbrella term for eye conditions of optic nerve neuropathy and that can lead to a loss of vision. The possible cause of damage to the optic nerve is excessive fluid pressure within the eye, which can be caused by increased aqueous production, blockage of drainage ducts and narrowing or closure of the iris angle. However, in normal tension glaucoma (NTG) the drainage angle for fluid within the eye is normal and IOP is within the normal range, but peripheral vision is lost. Essentially, glaucoma is a loss of homeostasis within the eye.

Glaucomatous optic neuropathy is the leading cause of irreversible blindness worldwide and the second-leading cause of overall blindness, following cataracts. About 70 million people have glaucoma globally, with about two million patients in the United States, with another two million who are undiagnosed! It is the leading cause of blindness in African Americans and it occurs more commonly among older people. Narrow-angle glaucoma is more common in women. Most sufferers have few or no symptoms of the disease, which occurs in 1 to 2 percent of the over-forty population. A family history of glaucoma or diabetes, a previous eye injury or surgery or the use of ocular steroids are considered risk factors for developing glaucoma.

The two aspects of glaucoma are: management of intraocular pressure and optic nerve health. Both of these issues must be addressed by any treatment protocol.

Intake of nutrients with antioxidant properties was examined in relation to open-angle glaucoma in the Nurses' Health Study and Health Professionals Follow-Up Study. No association was found. One small clinical trial found that supplementation with alpha-tocopherol (Vitamin E) for one year decreased markers of glaucomatous damage in patients with glaucoma. The authors suggested that alpha-tocopherol did not act through its antioxidant properties, but rather as a neuroprotective agent via regulatory mechanisms (e.g., inhibition of protein kinase C).

Studies of nutraceutical antioxidants including Ginkgo biloba, bilberry, red sage and lipoic acid have met with modest success in improving visual acuity and peripheral vision in people with glaucoma, possibly by improving circulation to the optic nerve. Elevated levels of homocysteine and depressed levels of folate, but not vitamin B12, were correlated with pseudoexfoliative glaucoma in one study. Another study found a beneficial relationship with supplements of vitamin B12.

There can be a problem of potency following ingestion with two particular supplements that have shown promise with glaucoma: CoQ10 and resveratrol. These have been shown to reduce mitochondrial susceptibility, and they show promise for neuroprotection.

One study found that topical micelles of CoQ10 with vitamin E (d-alpha-tocopherol) polyethylene glycol 1000 succinate, twice a day, significantly reduced the number of apoptotic retinal ganglion cells three weeks after induction of ocular hypertension. Furthermore, the effect was independent of IOP. Another study found that resveratrol retarded apoptosis of RGC's in vitro and decreased the level of a marker of apoptotic events, while stimulating increased quantities of mitochondria. Unfortunately, when a person ingests CoQ10 or resveratrol in supplement form, the efficacy may be dramatically altered by the metabolizing process. Clinical trials in humans could do a lot to pin down the quantities and concentrations required to produce similar effects in our patients.

A few herbal supplements are also believed to have positive effects on the eyes and glaucoma.

*Gingko biloba.* This is a well-known antioxidant used widely in Europe to treat breathing problems and Reynaud's phenomenon, which is a vascular disorder. Gingko is known to inhibit glutamate cytotoxicity, which leads to ganglion cell death, and it's been shown to increase blood flow. One of the challenges when studying gingko's effect on blood flow is that we still don't have agreement on the best way to measure ocular blood flow, making it difficult to draw any conclusions about how helpful gingko actually may be. One other important consideration when suggesting that a patient try gingko: Gingko increases the risk of bleeding. For that reason, you have to make sure your patient does not have wet AMD and is not on any blood thinners, because your patient could be prone to getting severe hemorrhages.

*Bilberry* (vaccinium myrtillus). The bilberry plant is a cousin of the blueberry. As an anthocyanidin, bilberry has a very potent antioxidant effect that can protect against ischemic reperfusion and neurotoxicity, and it's been shown to decrease retinal ganglion cell damage in a mouse model. However, no studies in humans have shown any effect on IOP or visual function. Bilberry is also a blood thinner so can interact with aspirin and warfarin and potentiate bleeding; and it has been associated with gastrointestinal upset, jaundice, cachexia and anemia.

*Forskolin* (coleus forskohlii). This herb has been shown to lower IOP in rabbits, monkeys and humans by reducing aqueous flow. However, studies were abandoned because forskolin caused significant hyperemia and tachyphylaxis. Furthermore, after a month or two the pressure would shoot back up, so there wasn't a lot of long-term promise. Oral preparations are available, but when you take forskolin orally it doesn't have any effect on IOP. Downsides include that forskolin is arrhythmogenic, and it can promote androgen activity on prostate cells in patients with prostate cancer.

*Cannabis* is commonly considered an "effective" alternative treatment for glaucoma. This is due to a 1971 study where it was reported that a 25 to 30% IOP lowering effect of smoking marijuana occurred in a small group. The proposal for action of the cannabinoids in the ocular tissue is that the effect occurs in both production and outflow of aqueous. This was a dose-response relationship lasting only 3-4 hours.

It does appear that marijuana can lower IOP for the management of glaucoma but the effects appear to be short-lived. To equal the sustainability of a typical topical prostaglandin the patient would have to consume or inhale the drug 6 to 8 times per day. There is evidence that there may be characteristics of the cannabinoid components of marijuana that are neuroprotective in nature. However, there are many other medications and nutrients that achieve this desired effect easier and with less euphoric side effect.

Intraocular inflammation, a significant risk factor in development of glaucoma, may be lessened by a combination of standardized bilberry extract and French maritime pine bark extract (as *Mirtogenol®*, containing 80 mg MirtoSelect® and 40 mg Pycnogenol®, (from Horphag Research). Italian researchers gave 38 individuals either Mirtogenol® or placebo for six months and measured intraocular pressure. At the end of the trial, they found intraocular pressure decreased in 19 of the 20 Mirtogenol® patients, compared to only one of the 18 patients in the control group. While the reduction in intraocular pressure was minimal, there was also a noted increase in optic nerve perfusion. Since glaucoma is actually an optic nerve disease, this finding should be considered significant.

*Nicotinamide riboside* (NR) is a member of the vitamin B3 family. It is found in small amounts in fruits, vegetables, meat, and milk. NR is changed in the body to a chemical called NAD+. NAD+ is essential for proper cell functioning and is involved in several metabolic activities, including protection against reactive oxygen species, contribution to the performance of various enzymes, and maintenance of mitochondrial function. It is also depleted with aging. Taking NR orally can help raise low NAD+ levels. This is not to be confused with niacin, niacinamide, or NADH. These are all related but are not the same.

Due to its beneficial effects and to the evidence of the reduction of NAD bioavailability with aging, researchers are seeking ways to replenish the cellular NAD pool, by administrating its precursors, believing that it will reduce the RGC vulnerability to external stressors, such as increased IOP.

A study was performed to determine the effects of oral administration of black currant anthocyanins (BCACs) on intraocular pressure in both healthy subjects and patients with glaucoma. A statistically significant decrease in the mean IOP was observed at 2 weeks and 4 weeks from the baseline in BCAC-treated healthy subjects. The results suggested that oral administration of BCACs may induce a beneficial decrease in IOP levels in healthy subjects as well as in patients with glaucoma.

Calcium (Ca), potassium (K) and magnesium (Mg) may be involved in the occurrence and development of glaucoma by influencing the retinal oxidative stress and regulate blood pressure. Data of 7,042 adults aged ≥40 years old who received the glaucoma examinations were extracted from the National Health and Nutrition Examination Survey (NHANES) database from 2005 to 2008 in this cross-sectional study. Enough dietary Ca, K, and Mg consumption may be potential protection factors of glaucoma that could provide some dietary reference for developing targeted glaucoma prevention and control measures.

*Nitric oxide* (NO) can increase aqueous humor outflow facility, inhibit aqueous humor production thereby reducing IOP, as well as regulate eye blood flow and protect the optic nerve. NO's ability to modulate the conventional aqueous humor outflow system, directly improving outflow through the trabecular meshwork, Schlemm's canal and distal scleral vessels.

*Capsanthin* is a carotenoid found in the Capsicum annuum species of plants including red bell pepper, New Mexico chiles, and cayenne peppers. This should not be confused with Capsaicin, the ingredient that creates the heat in chili peppers. It is one of the most potent carotenoids due to eleven conjugated double-bonds. It is also effective in reducing ocular surface inflammation. Results of a study showed that 28-day repeated administration of Capsanthin at dose levels of 20, 40 and 80 mg/kg reduced IOP from day 8 onwards. At the end of 28 day, the IOP returned to a level almost equal to the untreated group. Oral administration of capsanthin resulted in a significant reduction in IOP even at a low dose of 20 mg/Kg body weight.

One study demonstrated that *Pyrroloquinoline Quinone* (PQQ) is neuroprotective in two models of retinal ganglion cell degeneration. They identified an increased ATP content in healthy retinal ganglion cell-related contexts both in in vitro and in vivo models. Although PQQ administration resulted in a moderate effect on mitochondrial biogenesis and content, a metabolic variation in non-diseased retinal ganglion cell-related tissues was identified after PQQ treatment. These results suggest the potential of PQQ as a novel neuroprotectant against retinal ganglion cell death.

Large fluctuations in IOP during consecutive days (taken at approximately the same time of day) may be associated with allergy or food sensitivity. Allergy responses are known to cause altered vascular permeability and vasospasm, which could result in the congestion and edema found in glaucoma. In the trabecular network, histamine increases intracellular influx of calcium, increasing smooth muscle tension and potentially reducing circulation. Histamine has been shown to cause a reduction in the ability of the trabecular network cells to keep the meshwork clear of debris, resulting in increased IOP. Be sure to ascertain a complete case history from the patient regarding these issues.

Risk factors that affect glaucoma are generally those associated with vascular problems, including hypertension, hypotension, migraine, increased blood viscosity, carotid artery stenosis, and heart disease.

Prolonged stress and an inadequate diet over a long period of time are considered by many authorities to be the main causative factors in glaucoma. Prolonged stress leads to adrenal exhaustion, and exhausted adrenals are no longer able to produce aldosterone, which stabilizes the salt balance in the body. In this theory, when too much salt is lost from the body, the tissue fluids build up and often will push into the eyeball, increasing the intraocular pressure, forcing the lens forward. This closes off the anterior chamber, causing the pressure increase and damaging the optic nerve

Since one cause of glaucoma may be adrenal exhaustion, as discussed above, it is important to give the adrenal glands nutritional support. In general, any disturbance in the metabolism may lead to an increase in the eye pressure. Many of these supplements should be taken *with* any medication you prescribe.

Exercise has also been shown to be effective at reducing eye pressure. Researchers from the UCLA reported a 73 percent decline in the risk of developing the disease among the most physically active study participants, compared with those who were the least active. Studies on yoga have been mixed but, for the most part, be cautious of "inversion" postures with glaucoma patients. Be sure the patient checks with their primary healthcare provider before starting any exercise program.

| NUTRITIONAL SUPPLEMENTS | | |
|---|---|---|
| **Supplement** | **Directions for Use** | **Comments** |
| Acetyl-L-Carnitine | 500 mg daily | Neuroprotective |
| Black Currant Seed Oil | 50 mg daily | Excellent antioxidant |
| Capsanthin | 40 mg daily | Reduces IOP to normal levels |
| Choline and inositol | 1,000–2,000 mg of a combination supplement daily | Important B vitamins for the eyes |

| Supplement | Directions for Use | Comments |
|---|---|---|
| CoQ10 enzyme | 100 mg daily | Supports mitochondrial health |
| Fish oil | 2000 mg EPA/DHA daily | Has been shown to lower eye pressure; neuroprotection |
| Glutathione | 500 mg twice daily | A powerful antioxidant |
| Longevinex® | 364 mg daily | Anti-inflammatory |
| Manganese | 4 mg daily | An enzyme activator |
| Mirtogenol ® | 2 pills per day-morning and evening | Increases ocular perfusion |
| Nicotinamide Riboside | 300 mg daily | Reduces IOP |
| Niacin (Nicotinic Acid) | 30 mg daily | Shown to reduce risk of glaucoma |
| Rutin | 50 mg 3 times daily | Works with vitamin C to reduce the eye pressure |
| Vitamin A | 3,000 IU daily | Aids in mucopolysaccharide metabolism |
| Vitamin B3 | 300 mg daily | Supports neuroprotection |
| Vitamin B5 | 100 mg 3 times daily | A stress vitamin needed for the adrenal glands |
| Vitamin C | 2,000 mg daily-spread out evenly throughout day | Reduces the eye pressure |
| Vitamin E | 300-400 mg/daily | Increases blood flow to posterior ciliary arteries |

| HERBS AND HERBAL SUPPLEMENTS | | |
|---|---|---|
| **Herb** | **Directions for Use** | **Comments** |
| Bilberry | As directed on the label | Acts as an antioxidant |
| Er ming zuo ci wan (Boiron) | 8 pills 3 times daily or drink as a tea | Reduces congestion |
| Eyebright | Drink as a tea | Good for all eye conditions |

*(continued)*

| HERBS AND HERBAL SUPPLEMENTS (*con't*) | | |
|---|---|---|
| **Herb** | **Directions for Use** | **Comments** |
| Ginkgo Biloba and zinc sulfate | As directed on the label | Increases circulation |
| Ming mu di huang wan (Boiron) | 10 pills 3 times daily or drink as a tea | Clarifies the vision |
| Nei zhang ming yan wan (Boiron) | 8 pills 3 times daily | Clarifies the vision. *Caution:* Contains aluminum, so limit its use |
| Rose hips | Drink as a tea | A source of vitamin C |
| Shi hu ye guang wan (Boiron) | 1 pill twice daily | Reduces the eye pressure |

| HOMEOPATHIC REMEDIES | | |
|---|---|---|
| **Remedy** | **Directions for Use** | **Comments** |
| Belladonna 6c | 3–4 pellets under the tongue 3–4 times daily | Relieves the colored halo around lights |
| Nux vomica 6c | 3–4 pellets under the tongue 3–4 times daily | Good for high eye pressure |
| Phosphorus 6c | 3–4 pellets under the tongue 3–4 times daily | Relieves the colored halo around lights |
| Pulsatilla 6c | 3–4 pellets under the tongue 3–4 times daily | Relieves the colored halo around lights |
| Sulphur 6c | 3–4 pellets under the tongue 3–4 times daily | Good for glaucoma with pain |

## RECOMMENDATIONS FOR PATIENTS

- It is critical to have your eye pressure checked regularly to monitor the progress of your condition. Glaucoma often has no symptoms!
- Since the peripheral vision is affected first, be sure to have that tested periodically too.

- Be careful when drinking large amounts of fluids if glaucoma runs in the family. Moderate amounts are recommended.
- Avoid tobacco smoke, nicotine, alcohol, and all caffeine.
- Also, avoid consuming refined carbohydrates, such as white bread, which are taxing to the adrenal glands.

## GRAVE'S DISEASE

Grave's disease is one of the more common types of hyperthyroidism. It is a disorder in which the thyroid gland produces too much thyroid hormone, resulting in an overactive metabolism. All of the body's processes speed up, so the symptoms may include nervousness, irritability, a constant feeling of being hot, increased perspiration, insomnia, and fatigue. Patients often also present the symptoms of goiter (enlarged thyroid gland), exophthalmos (Thyroid Eye Disease, or TED), tachycardia, weight loss, hyperactive reflexes, drooping eyelids, and tremor. The thyroid gland may be normal sized in a small number of patients. The eye symptoms may include pain, excessive tearing, blurred vision, and diplopia.

The thyroid gland is the body's internal thermostat. It regulates the body's temperature by secreting two hormones that control how quickly the body burns calories and uses energy. Many cases of hyper- and hypothyroidism are believed to result from an abnormal immune response. The exact cause is not understood, but it is an autoimmune disorder where antibodies invade and attack the thyroid, disrupting the hormone production.

The age of onset of Grave's disease is most commonly between thirty and forty years old. Females are affected seven times more often than men.

### CONVENTIONAL TREATMENT

Grave's disease can be treated with medication or surgery. The surgery for Grave's disease involves the removal of thyroid tissue to reduce the overall hormone output to normal. Surgery, however, is not the preferred method of treatment because of the complications that may be caused by the general anesthesia and the possibility of nerve damage. Furthermore, too little or too much thyroid tissue frequently is removed.

The medications used to treat Grave's disease are called anti-thyroidal medications. These medications may also alter the thyroid–immune system mechanisms that are central to the cause of Grave's disease. They control the symptoms of hyperthyroidism in 90 percent of patients. Permanent remission is achieved in 10 to 30 percent of patients. Unfortunately, the relapse rates are high, many about 50 percent, even in patients who were treated for more than two years. The relapse rates are even higher, nearly 90 percent, in patients who were treated for less than two years.

The current advances in medical treatment including teprotumumab (Tepezza®), tocilizumab, rituximab and mycophenolate and the indications for their use in the management of active, moderate-to-severe TED. Tepezza reduces eye bulging and double vision. It also improves the signs and symptoms of TED, including eye pain, redness, and swelling.

The side effects of the anti-thyroidal medications include fever, rash, itching, and neutropenia (decrease in WBC count). Rare but serious side effects are arthritis, blood vessel inflammation, and hepatitis. The risk of side effects increases as the dose is increased.

## SELF-TREATMENT

Because Grave's disease is a metabolic disturbance, it is imperative that patients watch their diet closely. Be sure they eat plenty of broccoli, Brussels sprouts, cabbage, cauliflower, kale, mustard greens, peaches, pears, rutabagas, soybeans, spinach, and turnips. These foods help to suppress the production of thyroid hormone.

| NUTRITIONAL SUPPLEMENTS | | |
|---|---|---|
| **Supplement** | **Directions for Use** | **Comments** |
| Multi-vitamin and mineral complex | Take as directed on the label. | People with Grave's disease need increased amounts of all the vitamins and minerals. |
| Vitamin B complex | Take 50 mg 3 times daily with meals. | Benefits thyroid function. |

| Supplement | Directions for Use | Comments |
|---|---|---|
| Vitamin B | Take 50 mg twice daily. | Benefits blood formation and energy levels. |
| Vitamin B2 | Take 50 mg twice daily. | Necessary for the normal functioning of all the cells, glands, and organs. |
| Vitamin B6 | Take 50 mg twice daily. | An enzyme activator. Necessary for proper immune function and antibody production. |
| Capsanthin | Two caplets daily | Maintains eye moisture |

| HERBS AND HERBAL SUPPLEMENTS | | |
|---|---|---|
| **Herb** | **Directions for Use** | **Comments** |
| Alfalfa | Take as directed on the label. | A good source of vitamin K. Good for relaxation. |
| Burdock | Take as directed on the label. | A good source of iron. |
| Eyebright | Use as an eyewash. | Maintains the eye moisture. |
| Gotu kola | Take as directed on the label. | Good for relaxation. |
| Kelp | Take as directed on the label. | An infection fighter. |
| Licorice | Take as directed on the label. | Good for stress. |

| HOMEOPATHIC REMEDIES | | |
|---|---|---|
| **Remedy** | **Directions for Use** | **Comments** |
| Aconite 6c | Place 3–4 pellets under the tongue 3–4 times daily. | Good for anxiety. |
| Arsenicum album 6c | Place 3–4 pellets under the tongue 3–4 times daily. | Good for anxiety. |
| Belladonna 6c | Place 3–4 pellets under the tongue 3–4 times daily. | Good for restlessness. |

(*continued*)

| HOMEOPATHIC REMEDIES | | |
|---|---|---|
| **Remedy** | **Directions for Use** | **Comments** |
| Iodium 6c | Place 3–4 pellets under the tongue 3–4 times daily. | Restores iodine intake by the thyroid gland. |
| Thyroidium 6c (Boiron) | Place 3–4 pellets under the tongue 3–4 times daily. | Regulates the metabolism. |

## RECOMMENDATIONS FOR PATIENTS

- Be wary of treatment with radioactive sodium iodine, which is often recommended for this condition. It has been known to cause severe side effects.
- Do not rush into surgery. Instead, try to improve your diet first.
- To help with your eye symptoms, use eyewashes and artificial tears to maintain eye moisture. If the eyes dry out at night, lightly tape them closed using surgical paper tape.

# HEADACHE

The most common complaint among optometric patients is headache. It is very often the first sign of a vision-related problem. However, almost everyone experiences headache at one time or another. Common causes are stress, tension, anxiety, allergies, constipation, coffee consumption, hunger, sinus pressure, muscular tension, hormone imbalance, trauma, nutritional deficiency, alcohol consumption, drug use, smoking, fever, and, of course, eyestrain.

Experts estimate that about 90 percent of all headaches are tension headaches and 6 percent are migraines. Tension headaches, as the name implies, are caused by muscular tension. Migraines result from, most likely, a disturbance in the blood circulation to the brain. Another type of headache is the cluster headache. This is a severe, recurring headache that strikes about 1 million Americans.

Vision-related headaches most often are located toward the front of the head, although there are a few exceptions. They occur most often at the middle or end of the day, are not present upon awakening in the morning, and do not produce visual auras such as flashing lights. They often strike in a different pattern on the weekend than during the week, or not at all on the weekend. They also affect one side of the head more than they do the other, and may be accompanied by a number of more general symptoms.

Because of all the symptoms that accompany headaches, it is important that you obtain a thorough history from the patient to determine the type of headache suffered. They should be asked about the time of the headache's onset, location of the pain, frequency, duration, severity, and precipitating factors such as stress, certain foods, and medications. You should also note such associated signs and symptoms as nausea, vomiting, light sensitivity, and sound sensitivity.

The migraine headache is a disorder consisting of localized symptoms that may or may not be associated with actual headaches. Migraines have a number of phases that exhibit definite symptoms. The first is called the *prodromal* or premonitory phase, during which the patient might suffer irritability, depression, or light or sound sensitivity. These symptoms may show up as early as two days before the actual headache. The second phase is called the *aura* phase and consists of visual symptoms such as flashing lights, halos around lights, zigzagging of lines, and distortion of shapes and colors. This phase typically evolves over twenty minutes and is commonly, but not always, followed by the headache itself. The headache may throb, be located on one or both sides of the head, and last from four to seventy-two hours. The final phase is called the *post-dromal* phase, which can leave the patient washed out and exhausted.

Because migraine headaches have a visual aspect to them, eye doctors are often the first to be consulted. Light sensitivity, blurred vision, auras, blind spots, flashes of colored lights, tunnel vision, and other disorders are all possible visual effects of migraine headaches.

## CONVENTIONAL TREATMENT

The medical establishment has trained us to expect some type of medication to cure almost every malady. This is no truer than with the common headache. The largest selling over-the-counter medications in this country today are aspirin and the newer forms that include the non-steroidal anti-inflammatory drugs (NSAIDS), which form a billion-dollar business.

## SELF-TREATMENT

There are many options for self-treating a headache. Most of them involve discovering the source of the condition that led to the headache, then treating that condition. People who suffer from frequent headaches may be reacting to certain foods or food additives, such as wheat, chocolate, monosodium glutamate (MSG), sulfites, sugar, fermented foods (such as cheese, sour cream, and yogurt), alcohol, vinegar, or marinated foods. Other possible causes are anemia, bowel problems, brain disorders, teeth grinding, high blood pressure, low blood sugar, sinusitis, spinal misalignment, toxic overdose of vitamin A, deficiency of vitamin B, or a nose, throat, or a myriad of eye disorders. Some of the most common include hyperopia, astigmatism, binocular imbalance and, of course, "eyestrain".

One of the more common conditions associated with headaches these days is Computer Vision Syndrome (also called Digital Eyestrain). Since it is so prevalent today, it is covered in a separate section, earlier in this book.

Many times, lying down and remaining quiet for a short period of time will alleviate a headache, especially a tension headache. One might recommend a cold washcloth over the painful spot to reduce the excessive blood flow to the area.

| NUTRITIONAL SUPPLEMENTS | | |
|---|---|---|
| **Supplement** | **Directions for Use** | **Comments** |
| Bromelain | Take 500 mg as needed. | An enzyme that helps to regulate the inflammatory response. |
| Calcium | Take 1,500 mg daily. | Relieves muscular tension. |

| Supplement | Directions for Use | Comments |
|---|---|---|
| Coenzyme Q10 | Take 30 mg twice daily. | Improves tissue oxygenation. |
| Evening primrose oil | Take 500 mg 3–4 times daily. | Supplies essential fatty acids, which promote circulation. |
| Glucosamine sulfate | Take as directed on the label. | A natural alternative to aspirin and NSAIDs. |
| Magnesium | Take 1,000 mg daily. | Relieves muscular tension. |
| Potassium | Take 100 mg daily. | Maintains the proper balance between sodium and potassium. |
| Vitamin-B complex | Take 50 mg 3 times daily. | Good for nerve function. *Note:* It is better to take the entire B complex than just isolated B vitamins. |
| Vitamin C | Take 2,000–8,000 mg daily in divided doses. | A free-radical scavenger. Good for stress. |
| Vitamin E | Take 400 IU daily. | Boosts the circulation. |

| HERBS AND HERBAL SUPPLEMENTS | | |
|---|---|---|
| **Herb** | **Directions for Use** | **Comments** |
| Burdock | Take as directed on the label. | An excellent detoxifier. |
| Er ming zuo ci wan (Brion) | Take 8 pills 3 times daily. | Good for headaches accompanied by ear-ringing. |
| Fenugreek | Take as directed on the label. | Good for headache. |
| Feverfew | Take as directed on the label. | Good for headache. *Caution:* Do not use during pregnancy. |
| Goldenseal | Take as directed on the label. | Soothing for the tissues. *Caution:* Do not take internally for more than 1 week. Do not use during pregnancy. |

(*continued*)

| HERBS AND HERBAL SUPPLEMENTS (*con't*) | | |
|---|---|---|
| **Herb** | **Directions for Use** | **Comments** |
| Lavender | Rub essential oil on the temples. | Good for headaches accompanied by stomach upset. |
| Lobelia | Take as directed on the label. | Good for tension headaches. *Caution:* Do not take internally. |
| Long dan xie gan wan (Brion) | Take 6 pills twice daily. | Reduces inflammation and "heat." |
| Marshmallow | Take as directed on the label. | An anti-inflammatory. |
| Mint | Rub essential oil on the sore area. | Calms the nerves. |
| Niu huang shang qing wan (Brion) | Take 10 pills daily. | Reduces "heat" and toxins in the body. *Caution:* Do not use during pregnancy. |
| Qi ju di huang wan (Brion) | Take 8 pills 3 times daily or drink as a tea. | Good for headaches resulting from a "yin" deficiency. |
| Rosemary | Take as directed on the label. | Boosts the circulation. |
| Skullcap | Take as directed on the label. | Relieves spasm. |
| Thyme | Take as directed on the label. | Good for sinus headaches. |
| White willow bark | Take as directed on the label. | Good for pain. |
| Xiao yao wan (Brion) | Take 8 pills 3 times daily. | Good for a wide range of symptoms. |

| HOMEOPATHIC REMEDIES | | |
|---|---|---|
| **Remedy** | **Directions for Use** | **Comments** |
| Aconite 6c | Place 3–4 pellets under the tongue 3–4 times daily. | Good for throbbing headaches. |
| Arsenicum album 6c | Place 3–4 pellets under the tongue 3–4 times daily. | Good for head colds. |
| Belladonna 6c | Place 3–4 pellets under the tongue 3–4 times daily. | Good for colds, flu, sore throats, and similar problems. |
| Bryonia 6c | Place 3–4 pellets under the tongue 3–4 times daily. | Relieves pressure inside the head. |
| Gelsemium sempervirens 6c | Place 3–4 pellets under the tongue 3–4 times daily. | Good for headaches that form a band around the head. |
| Nux vomica 6c | Place 3–4 pellets under the tongue 3–4 times daily. | Good for headaches at the back of the head or over the eyes. Good for sharp pains and for eyestrain resulting from overwork. |
| Ruta graveolens 6c | Place 3–4 pellets under the tongue 3–4 times daily. | Supports the tendons and ligaments. |
| Sulphur 6c | Place 3–4 pellets under the tongue 3–4 times daily. | Relieves hot, burning sensations at the top of the head. |

## RECOMMENDATIONS TO PATIENTS

- Eat a well-balanced diet. Avoid chewing gum, ice cream, iced beverages, and salt.
- Avoid excessive sunlight.
- Practice deep-breathing exercises. A lack of oxygen can cause headaches.

- If you use a computer, take breaks often. For more treatments and recommendations, see the "Computer Vision Syndrome" section above.
- Always seek and treat the cause of a headache. Long-term reliance on aspirin and other painkillers can make chronic headaches worse by interfering with the brain's natural ability to fight them.

## HORDEOLUM

A stye looks and feels like a pimple on the edge of the eyelid—because that's what it is. It is often somewhat painful. You can differentiate a stye from a chalazion, by tugging slightly at the eyelid skin. If the pimple or swollen area moves *with* the skin, it's probably a stye. If the skin slides *over* the mass, it's likely a chalazion. Chalazia are most often painless. (For a complete discussion of chalazia, see previous section)

### CONVENTIONAL TREATMENT

Most styes go away within a week or so, but a stubborn one can be incised and drained. Topical antibiotics are also sometimes needed.

### SELF-TREATMENT

A stye can be brought to a head by steam bathing. You can also use a washcloth soaked in warm water or one of the herb teas listed below.

There are some over-the-counter remedies for styes that contain a compound called mercuric oxide. These remedies may work, but the mercury in these preparations can be very irritating to the eye. Mercury causes itching, stinging, and redness in many people. For this reason, most doctors don't recommend these products.

| NUTRITIONAL SUPPLEMENTS | | |
|---|---|---|
| **Supplement** | **Directions for Use** | **Comments** |
| Vitamin A | Take 5,000 IU daily. | Supports epithelial tissue. Especially beneficial if styes are a frequent problem. |
| Omega-3 EFAs | 2000 mg daily | Anti-bacterial; supports lid glands |

| HERBS AND HERBAL SUPPLEMENTS | | |
|---|---|---|
| **Herb** | **Directions for Use** | **Comments** |
| Eyebright | Apply as a compress or use as an eyewash. | Good for all eye conditions. |
| Raspberry | Apply as a compress or use as an eyewash. | Alleviates redness and irritation. |

## RECOMMENDATIONS TO PATIENTS

- Do not attempt to drain the head of a mature stye. Doing this can lead to more serious problems. Instead, contact our clinic for proper treatment.

# HYPERTENSIVE RETINOPATHY

Hypertensive retinopathy is a pathological condition of the retina directly caused by high blood pressure. Because of the extensive retinal vasculature, any condition that affects blood vessels can in turn affect the retina.

It is beyond the scope of this book to discuss all of the causes of hypertension, but it is certainly worth looking at how to control the disorder. Hypertension most often has no symptoms. The warning signs associated with advanced hypertension include headache, sweating, rapid pulse, shortness of breath, dizziness, and various visual disturbances.

Hypertension is usually divided into two categories—primary and secondary. Primary hypertension is high blood pressure that is not due to any other, underlying disorder. The precise cause of primary hypertension is unknown, but a number of definite risk factors have been identified. These include cigarette smoking, stress, obesity, and excessive use of stimulants such as coffee or tea, drug abuse, high sodium intake, and use of oral contraceptives.

Secondary hypertension is the result of another health problem, such as a hormonal abnormality or an inherited aortic stenosis. Secondary hypertension may also result from the blood vessels being chronically constricted or having lost their elasticity due to atherosclerosis. Atherosclerosis and arteriosclerosis (thickening of the artery walls) are common precursors of hypertension, and viewing the retinal blood vessels can assess both of these conditions.

## CONVENTIONAL TREATMENT

The standard treatment of hypertensive retinopathy is directed at both resolving the basic problem (the high blood pressure) and preventing the progression of the disease. Preventing the development of hypertension should be a primary goal of all persons at risk for the disease—that is, those persons with the risk factors discussed above or with a family history of the disease.

The first thing that must be done to treat hypertensive retinopathy is to recognize that the disorder exists. Signs of the condition can show up early in the disease process, so treatment of the disease can reduce the severity of the eye complications. Narrow arterioles and A/V niching are both signs of early disease.

There are more than a hundred different blood-pressure-lowering medications presently available. Most of these belong to six major classes—the beta blockers, diuretics, alpha blockers, calcium channel blockers, angiotensin-converting enzyme (ACE) inhibitors, and angiotensin antagonists. Within each class are several medications that are very similar to each other. Many physicians start with either a beta blocker or a diuretic because these are the medications that have been the most widely used in the trials demonstrating that lowering of the blood pressure reduces the risk of stroke and heart attack. In other words, they are the tried-and-true medications. Of the newer agents, the calcium channel blockers and ACE inhibitors are very popular, and may have fewer side effects. However, it remains to be seen if they are as good as the beta-blockers and diuretics at preventing stroke and heart attack.

Not every medication works well for every patient. It would be wonderful if the doctor could tell which medication will work the best with the least side effects, but unfortunately, no doctor can do this. There are some medications are contraindicated; beta-blockers, for example, make asthma worse. Beyond that, selecting the most appropriate medication is a hit-or-miss process.

Laser treatment is used on the retinal vessels to seal off the leakages. Usually, it is a spot laser treatment, which targets a specific point of leakage. The leakage is detected using fluorescein angiography. If there are several points of leakage, a scanning treatment (PRP) can be effective at targeting the multiple areas.

| NUTRITIONAL SUPPLEMENTS | | |
|---|---|---|
| **Supplement** | **Directions for Use** | **Comments** |
| Calcium and magnesium | Take 1,500–3,000 mg of a combination supplement daily. | Deficiencies have been linked to hypertension. |
| Coenzyme Q10 | Take 100 mg daily. | Improves heart function, and lowers blood pressure. |
| L-carnitine, L-glutamic acid, and L-glutamine | Take 500 mg of a combination supplement twice daily. Take on an empty stomach. | Help to prevent heart disease. |
| Lecithin | Take 1,200 mg 3 times daily. | Emulsifies fat in the body, and lowers blood pressure. |

(*continued*)

| NUTRITIONAL SUPPLEMENTS (*con't*) | | |
|---|---|---|
| **Supplement** | **Directions for Use** | **Comments** |
| Selenium | Take 100 mcg daily. | Deficiency has been linked to heart disease. |
| Vitamin C | Take 3,000–6,000 mg daily. | Improves adrenal function, and reduces blood clotting. |
| Vitamin E | Take up to 400 IU daily. | Improves heart function. |

| HERBS AND HERBAL SUPPLEMENTS | | |
|---|---|---|
| **Herb** | **Directions for Use** | **Comments** |
| Cayenne | Take as directed on the label. | Boosts the circulation. |
| Fennel | Take as directed on the label. | An anti-inflammatory. |
| Garlic | Take 250 mg 3 times daily. | Effective at lowering the blood pressure. |
| Hawthorn | Take as directed on the label. | Boosts the circulation. |
| Hops | Take as directed on the label. | Promotes relaxation of the smooth muscles. |
| Lady's slipper | Take as directed on the label. | Good for relaxation. |
| Parsley | Take as directed on the label. | Relieves mucous discharge. |
| Passion flower | Take as directed on the label. | Good for relaxation. |
| Rosemary | Take as directed on the label. | Stimulates the skin. |
| Scullcap | Take as directed on the label. | Relieves smooth-muscle spasm. |
| Valerian | Take as directed on the label. | Calms the nerves. |

| HOMEOPATHIC REMEDIES | | |
|---|---|---|
| **Remedy** | **Directions for Use** | **Comments** |
| Crataegus oxycantha 6c | Place 20 drops of tincture in 4 oz of water, and drink. Use daily for 3 months. | Regulates the blood pressure. |
| Lachesis 6c | Place 3–4 pellets under the tongue 3–4 times daily. | Increases vascular integrity. |
| Natrum muriaticum 6c | Place 3–4 pellets under the tongue 3–4 times daily. | Good for increased salt intake. |

## RECOMMENDATIONS TO PATIENTS

- Consider lifestyle counseling, a program to revamp your way of living. Lifestyle counseling will address your eating habits, exercise routine, stress level, work habits, and more.
- People with high blood pressure often have sleep apnea. If you have this condition, consult your physician.
- Avoid artificial sweeteners, which contain phenylalanine. Many contain warnings on their packages.
- Have your blood pressure checked at least every few months. If necessary, buy your own blood pressure checking equipment, available at most pharmacies.
- *Lose weight.* Of all the non-drug methods of lowering the blood pressure, losing weight is definitely the most effective. On average, a ten-pound loss of weight lowers the blood-pressure reading by as much as five points.
- *Exercise more.* Exercise helps partly by boosting the weight loss, but also is beneficial in its own right. The usual goal is at least thirty

minutes of aerobic exercise three times a week. Weightlifting and bodybuilding are not recommended.

- *If you are a regular drinker, cut down on your alcohol intake.* More than one or two drinks a day for men (one a day for women) raise the blood pressure.
- *Reduce your salt intake.* This doesn't work for everyone, and it is more likely to be effective if you are more than forty-five years old and have definite hypertension. In younger people and those with borderline hypertension, losing weight is much more important.
- *Increase your potassium intake.* Fruits and vegetables are good sources of potassium and are also low in sodium.
- *Try stress reduction.* In general, however, stress-reduction techniques such as biofeedback and relaxation have been found to be only marginally successful.
- *Quit smoking.* If you smoke, quitting may be the best thing you ever do. It won't have much effect on your blood pressure, but it will greatly reduce your risk of having a stroke or heart attack. Tobacco smoke will easily negate any of the positive recommendations a doctor can make.

## IRITIS

Iritis is an inflammation of the iris, and sometimes includes the ciliary body. The cause of iritis often is not known. Even when the disorder is treated early, it often recurs. In most cases, however, it eventually disappears completely.

In many cases, iritis is related to a disease or infection in another part of the body. Diseases such as arthritis, tuberculosis, or syphilis can contribute to its development. Infection in some organs such as the tonsils, sinuses, kidneys, gallbladder, or teeth can also cause inflammation of the iris. In other cases, iritis may follow an injury to the eye or accompany a corneal ulcer or foreign body. The symptoms of iritis usually appear suddenly and develop rapidly over a few hours or days. Iritis commonly causes extreme pain, redness, tearing, light sensitivity, and blurred vision. Some patients experience an increase in floaters.

A careful eye examination is extremely important when the symptoms of iritis occur. You may consider recommending blood tests, skin tests, and X-rays be conducted, and other specialists should be consulted to help determine the cause of the inflammation.

## CONVENTIONAL TREATMENT

The conventional treatment of iritis is often directed at finding and removing the cause of the inflammation. In addition, steroid drops and ointments are recommended to relieve the pain, quiet the inflammation, dilate the pupil, and reduce any scarring that may occur. Both steroids and antibiotics may be prescribed. In severe cases, oral medications and injections may be necessary.

A case of iritis usually lasts six to eight weeks. During this time, patients must be observed carefully for side effects from the medications and any complications. Cataracts, glaucoma, corneal changes, and secondary inflammation of the retina may occur as a result of the iritis or the medications.

The nutritional recommendations are listed to support your primary medical treatment of the condition.

| NUTRITIONAL SUPPLEMENTS | | |
|---|---|---|
| **Supplement** | **Directions for Use** | **Comments** |
| Boron | 3 mg daily | Supports the connective tissue. |
| Bromelain | As directed on the label | Assists in the production of prostaglandins. |
| Evening primrose oil | As directed on the label | Assist in the production of prostaglandins |
| Fish Oil | 3,000 mg EPA+DHA daily | Anti-inflammatory |

*(continued)*

| NUTRITIONAL SUPPLEMENTS | | |
|---|---|---|
| **Supplement** | **Directions for Use** | **Comments** |
| Superoxide dismutase (SOD) | As directed on the label | An antioxidant |
| Vitamin B5 | 500 mg daily | Vital for the production of steroid hormones |
| Vitamin E | 400 IU daily | An antioxidant |

| HERBS AND HERBAL SUPPLEMENTS | | |
|---|---|---|
| **Herb** | **Directions for Use** | **Comments** |
| Belladonna | As directed on the label | Dilates the pupil |
| Curcumin | 375 mg 3 times a day | Excellent anti-inflammatory |
| Cat's claw | As directed on the label | Good for pain. *Caution:* Do not use during pregnancy. |
| Feverfew and ginger | As directed on the label | Good for pain and soreness. *Caution:* Do not use feverfew during pregnancy. |

| HOMEOPATHIC REMEDIES | | |
|---|---|---|
| **Remedy** | **Directions for Use** | **Comments** |
| Aconite 6c | 3–4 pellets under the tongue 3–4 times daily | Good for iritis in the early stages |
| Allium cepa 6c | 3–4 pellets under the tongue 3–4 times daily | Good for inflammation |
| Apis mellifica 6c | 3–4 pellets under the tongue 3–4 times daily | Alleviates swelling |
| Belladonna 6c | 3–4 pellets under the tongue 3–4 times daily | Good for inflammation accompanied by dilated pupils |
| Calcarea fluorica 6c | 3–4 pellets under the tongue 3–4 times daily | Good for inflammation accompanied by light sensitivity |

| Remedy | Directions for Use | Comments |
|---|---|---|
| Euphrasia officinalis 6c | 3–4 pellets under the tongue 3–4 times daily | Good for all eye conditions |
| Mercurius corrosivus 6c | 3–4 pellets under the tongue 3–4 times daily | Alleviates pain and inflammation |
| Rhus toxicodendron 6c | 3–4 pellets under the tongue 3–4 times daily | Good for inflammation accompanied by muscle paralysis |

## RECOMMENDATIONS FOR PATIENTS

- If you are diagnosed with iritis, keep your eyes "quiet"—that is, avoid light, wind, dust, sun, and other types of irritations.

## MACULAR DEGENERATION

Age-related macular degeneration (AMD) is the second leading cause of blindness in the US. For one in four people over the age of sixty-five and for one in three over the age of eighty, the macula begins to degenerate. Very often, the macular area of one eye shows this degenerative change while the other eye remains perfectly normal. In this circumstance, patients may not notice any change taking place because the good eye will dominate the vision.

There are two forms of AMD—the wet and the dry forms. The wet form accounts for only 10 percent of cases. The dry form constitutes the other 90 percent of cases and occurs when drusen start to accumulate beneath the macula. These deposits gradually break down the photoreceptors in the macula, causing distorted vision in the affected eye, but is less severe than the vision loss in the wet variety.

There are certain risk factors that can increase one's susceptibility to AMD. These risk factors are:

–*Age.* It is estimated that about 14 percent of people aged fifty-five to sixty-four have some form of AMD. This rises to about 25 percent of persons aged sixty-five to seventy-five, and up to 37 percent of those over seventy-five.

–*Diet and nutrition.* The macula's fragile cells are highly susceptible to damage from free radicals. Research shows that people with a low dietary intake of antioxidants may be at risk for developing AMD. In addition, alcohol may deplete the body of antioxidants. High levels of saturated fats and fewer unsaturated fats harm blood vessels and are also involved in producing free-radical reactions.

–*Sunlight.* The cells of the macula are highly metabolic cells and damage from the sun can lead, over time, to deterioration of the macula. People with light colored eyes may be more prone to damage from sunlight than people with dark eyes. While the cornea and lens absorb UV light, blue light is the highest energy light reaching the retina. There is more blue light coming from the sun than any other source (including computer screens).

–*Smoking.* Recent studies showed that smoking, which reduces the protective antioxidants in the eye, more than doubles the risk of AMD. The studies have found that AMD is more than twice as common in people who smoke more than one pack of cigarettes a day than in people who do not smoke, and the risk remains high even up to fifteen years after quitting.

–*Heredity.* Some studies have shown that AMD may be in part inherited. This means that if someone has one or more immediate relatives with AMD, they may be at a higher risk for developing the condition.

–*Gender and race.* Women over the age of seventy-five have double the chance of developing AMD as men of the same age. Low levels of estrogen in postmenopausal women may also increase the risk for the condition. There is some suggestion that postmenopausal estrogen therapy may protect against AMD, but more research is needed in this area. Women also live longer than men. Caucasians are much more likely than African-Americans to lose vision to AMD.

*–Heart disease.* If you have high blood pressure or another form of heart disease, you may also have a greater chance of getting AMD because of the poor blood circulation to the eyes.

Macular degeneration does not result in total blindness but since only the macular area is affected, a person afflicted with macular degeneration can feel very helpless and frustrated due to the loss of detail vision. The peripheral vision usually remains intact and therefore allows the person to function almost normally. This is especially true if only one eye is affected.

## CONVENTIONAL TREATMENT

At one time lasers had been used in the treatment of the wet form of macular degeneration. In this procedure, the laser was used to coagulate the leaking vessels near the macula. However, this most often resulted in a significant loss of visual acuity.

More recent developments in the medical treatment of AMD have focused on the wet form. The first approved treatment of AMD was called Photo-Dynamic Therapy (PDT). This process used a photosensitive compound called verteporfin. This drug is injected into the bloodstream and it traveled to the retina, where it was then activated by shining a low intensity laser onto the damaged area. This causes a chemical reaction that destroys the abnormal blood vessels. While it is effective in retarding the deterioration of vision, it had to be repeated several times a year and vision was also lost.

In 2004, genetic research discovered the Vascular Endothelial Growth Factor, or VEGF. It was also determined that this factor was responsible for the growth of the blood vessels in the macula secondary to AMD. This has led to research to develop medications that inhibit this blood vessel growth factor (thus the category name, "Anti-VEGF" drugs).

The first of these medications is called Macugen (pegaptanib sodium). Macugen worked by blocking an essential signal that causes abnormal blood vessels to grow and leak. Macugen was not a cure, but it helped to slow further vision loss and also to help preserve vision. Macugen treatment required intraocular injections about every 4-6 weeks.

A second treatment in this category is called Lucentis (ranibizumab). It also inhibited blood vessel growth, thereby preventing scar tissue development and protecting vision.

A third drug, called Avastin was not approved for use on AMD. It was prescribed for metastatic colorectal cancer, but has been used "off-label" in the eye. It has been effective in halting the progression of AMD and was eventually approved as a drug for AMD.

Since then, several newer drugs have been developed, each with an advancement of the treatment of the disease. Vabysmo, Eyelea (and EyeleaHD), Syfovre (for geographic atrophy) are all being used in the treatment for late dry and wet AMD.

However, the earlier forms of macular degeneration cannot yet be reliably treated either medically or surgically. The best way to "treat" AMD is prevention.

## SELF-TREATMENT

The largest study of nutritional treatment for AMD was concluded in the late 1990s. This study was called the Age-Related Eye Disease Study, or AREDS. The supplement that the study participants took was a combination of beta carotene (15mg); Vitamin C (500mg); Vitamin E (400 IU); Zinc Oxide (80 mg) and Copper Oxide (2 mg). The result showed that while there was no preventive effect nor was there any reversal of AMD, there was a slowing of the progression from stage III to stage IV (the most advanced stages). The product is marketed as Preservision® (B+L). There are several concerns with the study protocol since almost ⅔ of the study subjects were already taking a multi-vitamin of some form and that they were allowed to continue to take their vitamins during the study. Also, the amount of zinc in this formula is well over the RDA allowance of daily zinc intake, so caution should be taken with this formula.

In 2006, a follow-up study, called AREDS2 published their results. This formula was similar to AREDS but it also substituted lutein and zeaxanthin for beta-carotene and considered lower amounts of zinc. While there are some benefits to recommending the AREDS2 formula, there are many more nutrients that can affect macular function that are detailed in the charts below. Here is a comparison of the two studies:

| AREDS 1 | AREDS 2 |
|---|---|
| **Formula:**<br>Vitamin C (500 mg)<br>Vitamin E(400 IU)<br>Beta-carotene (15 mg)<br>Zinc (80 mg as zinc oxide)<br>Copper (1 mg as copper oxide) | **Formula:**<br>Vitamin C (500 mg)<br>Vitamin E (400 IU)<br>Lutein (10 mg)<br>Zeaxanthin (2 mg)<br>Zinc (80 mg as zinc oxide)<br>Copper (2 mg of cupric oxide) |
| Younger: average age 69 | Older: average age 74 |
| All stages of AMD | Sicker- stages 3 and 4 only |
| Typical SAD diet | "Well-nourished" |
| Diabetes: 7% | Diabetes: 13 % |
| Centrum Silver (no lutein): 67% | Centrum Silver (with lutein): 89% |
| Demographic- unclear | Few Hispanics (2%) |

While patients cannot change their age, sex, or family tree, there are some lifestyle changes that can be adopted to help protect vision. First, wear sunglasses or a brimmed hat whenever exposed to large amounts of UV light. Moderate amounts of UV light are good for the human body, but overexposure can cause damage to the eye.

Anything that prevents arterial blockage may help to prevent macular degeneration. Therefore, watching the dietary sugar and simple carbohydrate intake, exercising regularly, not smoking, and watching weight and blood pressure are wise moves. Limiting intake of alcohol to a maximum of six drinks per week for men and three per week for women.

There have been reports that the BMI affects the amount of lutein and zeaxanthin in the retina. What this means is that the higher amount of body fat you have, the less is available for the retina. It seems that these nutrients are stored in fat tissue and are not available to the eye, even when needed.

Finally, most doctors recommend that their older patients take antioxidant supplements to prevent or halt the progress of macular degeneration. Recent studies indicate that a well-rounded combination of antioxidants can slow macular degenerative changes. Several research studies on AMD are focusing on the role of retinal carotenoids. Lutein and zeaxanthin are the only pigments found in the macula. By contrast, beta-carotene is virtually absent from the eye. Lutein and zeaxanthin can be found in almost all fruits and vegetables, but are most likely to be present in dark green leafy vegetables such as spinach, eggs and kale. Review the section of this book on Carotenoids for a full description.

| NUTRITIONAL SUPPLEMENTS | | |
|---|---|---|
| **Supplement** | **Directions for Use** | **Comments** |
| Selenium | Take 400 mcg daily. | An antioxidant. |
| Vitamin A | Take 10,000 IU daily. | An antioxidant. *Note:* Use the emulsion form for easier assimilation and greater safety. |
| Vitamin C with bioflavonoids | Take 1,000–2,500 mg 4 times daily. | An antioxidant. *Note:* Use powdered buffered ascorbic acid. |
| Vitamin E | Take 600–800 IU daily. | An antioxidant and free-radical scavenger. |
| Glutathione | 500 mg twice daily | Master antioxidant |
| Longevinex® | 350 mg daily | Good for retinal health |
| Lutein | 20 mg daily | Increases macular pigment |
| Zeaxanthin | 5 mg daily | Increases macular pigment |
| Zinc | Take 40 mg daily. | Deficiency has been linked to eye problems. *Caution:* Do not take more than 80 mg daily. *Note:* Use the zinc picolinate form. |

| HERBS AND HERBAL SUPPLEMENTS | | |
|---|---|---|
| **Herb** | **Directions for Use** | **Comments** |
| Bilberry | Take 160 mg daily. | Improves retinal function. |
| Blueberry | Drink 8–10 oz of tea daily. | Rich in flavonoids. |
| Ginkgo biloba | Take as directed on the label. | The dry form stimulates blood flow in the capillaries. Not for wet AMD! |

| HOMEOPATHIC REMEDIES | | |
|---|---|---|
| **Remedy** | **Directions for Use** | **Comments** |
| Hamamelis virginiana 6c | Place 3–4 pellets under the tongue 3–4 times daily. | Alleviates venous congestion and vascular infiltration. |
| Lachesis 6c | Place 3–4 pellets under the tongue 3–4 times daily. | Good for macular degeneration with muscle fatigue. |
| Phosphorus 6c | Place 3–4 pellets under the tongue 3–4 times daily. | Good for many eye conditions. Improves tissue metabolism, and reduces vascular and blood degeneration. |

## RECOMMENDATIONS TO PATIENTS

- While you can't stop the aging process, you can watch your diet. Eat a low-carb diet with lots of fresh vegetables and fruits, and a minimum of processed foods.
- Increase your consumption of legumes; yellow vegetables; flavonoid-rich berries, such as blueberries, blackberries, and cherries; and foods rich in vitamins C and E, such as raw fruits and vegetables.

- Avoid alcohol, cigarette smoke, all sugars, excessive saturated fats, and foods containing fats and oils that were subjected to heat or exposed to the air, such as fried foods, hamburgers, luncheon meats, and roasted nuts.
- If using blue-blocking lenses, have the blue-blocking technology in your sunglasses!

## MULTIPLE SCLEROSIS

Multiple sclerosis (MS) is an inflammatory disease of the body's central nervous system. This disease—which may, it is now believed, originate with a viral infection—destroys the myelin sheaths surrounding nerves. Another theory is that MS is an autoimmune disease in which white blood cells attack the myelin sheaths.

Early symptoms of multiple sclerosis (MS) can vary widely and may be subtle or intermittent. Some common early symptoms include: Numbness or tingling in the limbs, face, or trunk, weakness in the extremities, pins and needles sensation, heat or cold sensitivity, difficulty walking or coordinating movements, clumsiness or unsteadiness, and muscle stiffness or spasms.

Multiple sclerosis can affect the optic nerve itself, causing poor vision ranging from mild symptoms to changes in color vision, blind spots, and blindness. It can also affect the extraocular muscles causing double vision from strabismus, poor binocular coordination, and nystagmus. Very often, these visual problems are the first symptoms of MS.

MS is usually diagnosed between the ages of twenty-five and forty. Women are affected nearly twice as often as men. MS is rarely diagnosed in children and in people over sixty years of age. An MRI may be used to diagnose MS. However, there is no single diagnostic test for the disease, and diagnosis must be done indirectly, by ruling out other possible causes of the symptoms.

## CONVENTIONAL TREATMENT

Fortunately, most people with MS have periods of remission during which their symptoms improve or even disappear. Many years can go by before serious visual impairment occurs—and it doesn't occur at all in some patients. Systemic steroids and other medications are now used to improve the symptoms of multiple sclerosis, including the eye problems.

There is no known cure for MS, but the following supplement and dietary recommendations have been shown to be helpful. Long-term sufferers of MS may not benefit as much, but younger people who are just starting to exhibit symptoms may find that the correct supplements slow or even stop the progression of the disease.

| NUTRITIONAL SUPPLEMENTS | | |
|---|---|---|
| **Supplement** | **Directions for Use** | **Comments** |
| Choline and inositol | Take as directed on the label. | Stimulate the central nervous system, and protect the myelin sheaths from damage. |
| Coenzyme Q10 | Take 100 mg daily. | Boosts the circulation, and improves tissue oxygenation. Strengthens the immune system. |
| Evening primrose oil, gamma linolenic acid (GLA), or omega-6 oils | Take as directed on the label 3 times daily with meals. | All of these are essential fatty acids that can help to control MS symptoms. Deficiency is common in MS. |
| Sulfur | Take 500 mg 2–3 times daily. | Protects against toxic substances. |
| Vitamin-B complex | Take 100 mg 3 times daily. | Aids immune function, and maintains healthy nerves. |
| Vitamin B6 | Take 50 mg 3 times daily. | Promotes red blood cell production, and aids nervous-system and immune function. |

*(continued)*

| NUTRITIONAL SUPPLEMENTS | | |
|---|---|---|
| **Supplement** | **Directions for Use** | **Comments** |
| Vitamin B12 | Take 1,000 mcg twice daily. | Aids cellular longevity, and prevents nerve damage by maintaining the myelin sheaths. *Note:* Use the sublingual form. |
| Vitamin D | 5,000 IU daily | Acts like a hormone; provides nerve protection |

| HERBS AND HERBAL SUPPLEMENTS | | |
|---|---|---|
| **Herb** | **Directions for Use** | **Comments** |
| Alfalfa | Take as directed on the label. | A good source of vitamin K. |
| Burdock, dandelion, Echinacea, goldenseal, red clover, St. John's Wort, sarsaparilla, taheebo, and yarrow | Take as directed on the label. | All of these are excellent detoxifiers. |
| Garlic | Take 1,000 mg 3 times daily. | An excellent source of sulphur. |
| Lobelia, skullcap, and valerian | Take as directed on the label at bedtime. | Calm the nerves, and prevent insomnia. |

| HOMEOPATHIC REMEDIES | | |
|---|---|---|
| **Remedy** | **Directions for Use** | **Comments** |
| Aurum 6c | Place 3–4 pellets under the tongue 3–4 times daily. | Good for pain. |
| Hyoscyamus 6c | Place 3–4 pellets under the tongue 3–4 times daily. | Relieves spasm. |
| Natrum muriaticum 6c | Place 3–4 pellets under the tongue 3–4 times daily. | Good for pain. |
| Nitricum acidum 6c | Place 3–4 pellets under the tongue 3–4 times daily. | Good for pain. |

## RECOMMENDATIONS FOR PATIENTS

- A strong immune system may help to prevent the development of multiple sclerosis by assisting the body in avoiding infection, which often precedes the onset of the disease.
- Eat only organically grown foods that have not been chemically treated and contain no chemical additives, including eggs, fresh fruits, gluten-free grains, raw nuts and seeds, fresh vegetables, and cold-pressed vegetable oils.
- The best diet for people with multiple sclerosis is vegetarian.
- Eat plenty of raw sprouts and alfalfa, plus foods that contain lactic acid, such as sauerkraut and dill pickles. Also, green drinks, which contain plenty of chlorophyll, are good, as are dark green leafy vegetables. These are good sources of vitamin K.

## MYOPIA

Within the eyecare community, there is a predominant consensus that the cause of juvenile onset myopia involves both genetic and environmental elements. The rise in the prevalence of myopia has been too rapid to be explained by genetic factors alone and thus suggests a substantial role of environmental influences. However, the interaction of these two components to create refractive error remains speculative. It is becoming more apparent that myopia is not just a benign refractive error but has long term medical and visual consequences. Yet, little attention has been paid to the possible role of nutrition in the development and advancement of myopia.

Numerous studies have demonstrated that near point work is related to myopia. However, all people in industrialized countries must do regular near work during childhood education, yet only a certain percentage of the population ultimately develop myopia.

When considering the genetic influence on ocular growth and function, it must be considered to first look to our ancestral genetic makeup. Early Homo sapiens lived about 160,000 years ago and are considered to be an anatomically modern Homo sapiens. We can infer that significant myopia was not likely present in the population since these early humans required clear distance vision to escape predators, find food, recognition of other species members and a host of environmental dangers. Thus, any gene or genes that would produce high myopia would be lethal and rapidly eliminated by natural selection.

The diets of hunter-gatherer civilizations are typically considered high protein, moderate levels of fat and low levels of carbohydrate when compared to modern Western diets. Additionally, the carbohydrates present in hunter-gatherer diets were typically of a low glycemic index (see below). They are slowly absorbed and produce a gradual and minimal rise in plasma, glucose and insulin levels when compared to the sugars and refined starches in modern western diets.

The Glycemic Index (GI) is a ranking of carbohydrates on a scale from 0 to 100 according to the extent to which they raise blood sugar levels after eating. High GI Foods are those which are rapidly digested and absorbed and result in marked fluctuations in blood sugar levels. Low GI foods, by virtue of their slow digestion and absorption, produce gradual rises in blood sugar and insulin levels, and have proven benefits for health. The glycemic index is a measure influenced by the particle size, processing technique, and relative fiber protein and fat content of a carbohydrate food. A glycemic index of over 70 is consider high, 55-70 is medium and lower than 55 is low. A review of this rating system can be seen at: www.glycemicindex.com

The Glycemic Load (GL), which is a function of the net carbohydrate intake and its glycemic index, estimates how much a food raises a person's blood glucose level following its consumption. It is calculated by taking the glycemic index x carb content/100 of each food. For example, a high glycemic food like watermelon (index=72) only contains 11 net carbohydrates, thus has a GL of only 8, whereas white rice (index=64) contains 52 net carbohydrates and has a GL of 33. A glycemic load of 20 or higher is considered high. See the Glycemic Load chart in the chapter on Diets

The average glycemic load of foods of industrialized countries has continually increased, primarily from consumption of refined cereals and sugars. Populations in more rural areas of both industrialized and non-industrialized countries typically have limited access to these processed foods, sugars and refined cereal products. Accordingly, their diets are usually comprised of locally grown, minimally processed foods, and hence, the glycemic load of these traditional foods is generally lower than highly processed and packaged food.

Studies suggest that high glycemic load carbohydrate diets may alter the genetic influence of growth of the sclera and choroid which will in turn induce permanent changes in the development and progression of myopia, particularly during periods of growth. Collagen content in the sclera is significantly reduced during myopia development, with thinning of fibrils, loss of a fiber thickness gradient, and overall reduction in scleral thickness.

## CONVENTIONAL TREATMENT

Some of the more common treatments for myopia are:

- Orthokeratology- using reverse geometry gas permeable lenses to flatten the cornea and reduce refractive error.
- Soft contact lenses- Several companies have developed multifocal soft contact lenses to slow myopia progression, including MiSight; NaturalVue MF; Biofinity MF; Acuvue Oasys Presbyopia
- Spectacle lenses: Essilor Stellest® (using concentric rings of treatment zones in the lens that create an extra defocus signal)
- Low dose atropine - .0125% seems to be the most effective concentration
- Surgical intervention– Posterior scleral reinforcement (worst case scenario)

## SELF-TREATMENT

There is no escape from activities that require near-point focus. Consider all the things we do with our eyes at the near point—reading, writing, drawing, typing, painting, sewing, crocheting, and even cooking and eating, to name just a few. And then there are those intermediate-distance tasks, such as playing the piano (and most musical instruments), shopping, working at computers, card playing, watching television, and enjoying a variety of hobbies. During the grade-school years, children read the equivalent of about 700 books. When this reading time is added to play time and computer time, it's not hard to see why so many people develop myopia.

Several years ago, during a period of radio and TV promotions for the effects of excessive computer display use on the visual system, the author created the "3-B" approach to reduce eyestrain for display users. The process was to BLINK, BREATHE and BREAK! It was confirmed that we blink less while viewing a computer display and the eyes will dry and become uncomfortable. Breathing techniques will help to reduce stress for those employees with tight deadlines and computer programmers who have strict work requirements. For taking breaks, the author created the "20-20-20" rule, whereby a display user would take a 20-second break every 20-minutes and look away at a target 20-feet away. This was more of a "practical suggestion" than confirmed science. However, it was based on a study that confirmed that shorter, more frequent breaks were more beneficial than longer breaks at longer intervals. Given that it was promoted by an eyecare professional, it was easy to remember and rang true for many consumers.

Vision therapy is another alternative for myopia. However, it is more difficult to reverse myopia than it is to prevent it. You must dedicate yourself to your vision therapy program, and do all of the required techniques on a regular basis. Changing the visual process is a monumental task, but one may be able to do it if commit to the process and followed through completely.

Review the "Myopia Diet" in the last section of this book.

| NUTRITIONAL SUPPLEMENTS | | |
|---|---|---|
| **Supplement** | **Directions for Use** | **Comments** |
| Calcium | Take 800 mg daily | Important in collagen formation |
| Chromium | Take 30–100 mg daily | Deficiencies have been found in persons with myopia |
| Copper | Take 1 mg daily | Important in collagen formation |
| Vitamin A | Take 5,000 IU daily | Good for all eye conditions |
| Vitamin C | Take 1,000 mg three times daily | Strengthens the collagen for stronger eyes |
| Vitamin D | 5,000 IU daily | Affects cell signaling for eye growth |

| HERBS AND HERBAL SUPPLEMENTS | | |
|---|---|---|
| **Herb** | **Directions for Use** | **Comments** |
| Ming mu shang qing pian (Boiron) | Take 4 pills twice daily | Clarifies the vision. *Caution:* Do not use during pregnancy |

## RECOMMENDATIONS FOR PATIENTS

- Have complete eye exams regularly. This is especially important for school-aged children. Make sure that near vision abilities are tested.
- When doing a near-point activity, take regular breaks to give your eyes a rest. Follow the 20-20-20 rule (as above)
- Increase your intake of fiber, and reduce your intake of simple carbohydrates and sugars Avoid most processed foods.
- If you are sick with a fever, avoid near-point activities. High temperatures weaken and soften the collagen, which can easily become stretched with increased eye pressure.

## NIGHT BLINDNESS

*See* Nyctalopta.

## NYCTALOPIA

True night blindness is a relatively rare condition in the United States. The main symptom of this disorder is a decrease in visual acuity under nighttime viewing conditions. Most often, night blindness is caused by a nutritional deficiency—specifically, vitamin A—and is common in underdeveloped countries. Vitamin A is necessary for the formation of the rhodopsin required by the retina to transmit the nerve impulse that is responsible for vision. Other causes of night blindness are fatigue, nutritional deficiency, emotional disturbances, and hereditary factors.

It is also very common for persons who are just beginning to become myopic to complain of difficulty seeing clearly at night. This is different than true night blindness. It would be beneficial to explain to patients that the eyes generally become more myopic at night. In fact, night driving is one of the most challenging tasks we perform with our eyes. In addition, our eyes are usually more fatigued after being used all day long in stressful situations, thus leading to a poorer focusing ability. When the sunlight dims, the pupil dilates creating a myopic blur.

### CONVENTIONAL TREATMENT

The treatment for night blindness depends on the cause of the problem. For the simple problem of myopia, glasses are normally prescribed, often just for night driving. If a computer-using patient eyes are temporarily myopic but merely overstressed, you may advise them to use reading glasses for daily near-point activities. These will allow the eyes to relax more during close work and therefore keep them from being stressed for night viewing.

For the serious diseases such as retinitis pigmentosa, there are no conventional treatments available. However, new research is showing that nutritional supplementation might have a slowing effect on the progression of the disease.

## SELF-TREATMENT

The best thing that patients can do is to make an appointment for a full eye examination, which should include testing at the near viewing distance. Consider what alternatives are available for their condition. In general, supplementing your diet with vitamin A will help to protect your eyes against night blindness. Also, vitamins B1, B2, and B3, as well as zinc have been reported to relieve night blindness when vitamin A did not produce a response.

| NUTRITIONAL SUPPLEMENTS | | |
|---|---|---|
| **Supplement** | **Directions for Use** | **Comments** |
| Vitamin A | Take 10,000 IU daily. | Supports the retina. |
| Vitamin-B complex | Take 75–100 mg daily. | Good for nerve function. |
| Bilberry | 50 mg daily | Important for night vision |
| Copper | Take 1 mg daily | Must be used if zinc is taken |
| Lutein | 20 mg daily | Supports macular pigment |
| Zeaxanthin | 4 mg daily | Supports macular pigment |
| Zinc | Take 40 mg daily. | Good in combination with vitamin A. |

| HERBS AND HERBAL SUPPLEMENTS | | |
|---|---|---|
| **Herb** | **Directions for Use** | **Comments** |
| Eyebright | Take as directed on the label. | Good for all eye conditions |
| Qi ju di huang wan (Brion) | Take 8 pills 3 times daily or drink as a tea. | Aids liver function. |

## RECOMMENDATIONS TO PATIENTS

- Have a complete eye examination once a year.

- Regular examinations can catch night blindness before it becomes disabling.
- If doing excessive computer viewing, follow the "20-20-20" rule to relax accommodative stress

## OPTIC NEURITIS

Optic neuritis, also known as retrobulbar neuritis, Another line of research has is an inflammation of the optic nerve. Symptoms of optic neuritis include an acute blurring, graying, or loss of vision, almost always in one eye, although occasionally in both eyes. The visual deficit usually reaches its maximum within a few days, and generally improves within eight to twelve weeks.

Optic neuritis typically presents with a triad of symptoms—loss of vision, disturbed color vision, and eye pain. The initial attack is in just one eye in 70 percent of adult patients and in both eyes in 30 percent. The mean age of onset of the disorder is the twenties, but it can develop anytime from birth through the sixties. The annual incidence of optic neuritis ranges from 1.4 to 6.4 new cases per 100,000 people.

The visual loss accompanying optic neuritis can be subtle or profound. In some cases, the vision may be 20/20 with the only symptom being blurring upon exertion. The rate of visual decline varies. The visual loss can occur over a period of hours (rarely) to days (most commonly). The peak visual loss most often is about one week after the onset of the disorder. The prognosis for visual recovery usually is good. The majority of patients (65 to 80 percent) recover a visual acuity of 20/30 or better. Most patients recover their visual acuity within a few months, although they often report some residual visual defects. These residual defects have included decreased contrast sensitivity, disturbed color vision, visual field constriction, and light sensitivity.

It has been estimated that about half of patients with multiple sclerosis (MS) have an episode of optic neuritis. Frequently, optic neuritis is the first symptom of MS. While estimates of the subsequent development of MS in a person who presents with optic neuritis vary, studies with up to ten years of follow-up have demonstrated that approximately 50 to 60 percent of patients with isolated optic neuritis go on to develop MS. A more recent study reported that persons with optic neuritis who also had abnormalities in their spinal fluid were more likely to develop MS. Other studies have demonstrated that a majority of patients with optic neuritis have evidence of demyelination in the brain, as evidenced on MRI scanning. While other disease processes can cause optic neuritis, in a young, otherwise healthy person, MS is the most likely cause.

## CONVENTIONAL TREATMENT

Recent studies suggest that a short course of intravenous steroids followed by a tapered course of oral steroids may be useful in helping to reverse and restore vision damaged by optic neuritis, although there is no definitive evidence that treatment with steroids effects a more complete recovery than no treatment at all.

## SELF-TREATMENT

When a B-complex or B1 deficiency is responsible for the optic neuritis, supplementing with these vitamins will result in recovery within three to four days. The B vitamins must be taken in adequate amounts even when a deficiency doesn't exist, however, since they are needed for the general health of nerve tissue.

A well-balanced diet is important for the maintenance and repair of the muscles and nerves. Whenever there is an infection, patients should boost their protein, calorie, and fluid intakes.

| NUTRITIONAL SUPPLEMENTS | | |
|---|---|---|
| **Supplement** | **Directions for Use** | **Comments** |
| Essential fatty acids | 1,000 to 2,000 mg daily | Repair and rebuild the nerves. |
| Glutathione | Take 500–1,000 mg daily. | Supports the nerve and brain tissues. |

*(continued)*

| NUTRITIONAL SUPPLEMENTS | | |
|---|---|---|
| **Supplement** | **Directions for Use** | **Comments** |
| Lecithin | Take 2 tbsp twice daily. | Protects and repairs the nerves. *Note:* Use the granular form. |
| Magnesium | Take 400 mg daily. | Helps the body to utilize the B-complex vitamins. |
| Protein | Take .5 gm for every 1 lb of body weight daily. | Important for the repair of body tissues. |
| Vitamin-B complex | Take at least 100 mg daily. | Good for nerve function. |

| HERBS AND HERBAL SUPPLEMENTS | | |
|---|---|---|
| **Herb** | **Directions for Use** | **Comments** |
| Bilberry | Take 60 mg daily. | An antioxidant. |
| Oats | Take as directed on the label. | Calms the nerves. Soothing for the mucous membranes. |
| Skullcap | Take as directed on the label. | Calms the nerves, and relieves spasm. |
| St. John's wort | Take as directed on the label. | An anti-inflammatory. Repairs and rebuilds the nerves. |
| Valerian | Take as directed on the label. | Calms the nerves, and relieves spasm. |

| HOMEOPATHIC REMEDIES | | |
|---|---|---|
| **Remedy** | **Directions for Use** | **Comments** |
| Aconite 6c | Place 3–4 pellets under the tongue 3–4 times daily. | Good for optic neuritis in the early stages. Good for pain and inflammation. |
| Apis mellifica 6c | Place 3–4 pellets under the tongue 3–4 times daily. | Good for inflammation. |

| | | |
|---|---|---|
| Hypericum perforatum 6c | Place 3–4 pellets under the tongue 3–4 times daily. | Reduces nerve irritability. |
| Phosphorus 6c | Place 3–4 pellets under the tongue 3–4 times daily. | Good for many eye conditions. |
| Spigelia 6c | Place 3–4 pellets under the tongue 3–4 times daily. | Good for pain and nerve sensitivity. |

## RECOMMENDATIONS TO PATIENTS

- Relaxation is a key component of the healing process. Reduce the stress level in all the areas of your life.
- Avoid stimulants such as coffee, carbonated beverages, and cigarettes.
- Increase your fluid intake.
- Eat a diet of fresh fruits and vegetables, raw nuts and seeds, and whole grains.

# PINGUECULA

The word pinguecula comes from the Latin word for "fatty." A pinguecula is a yellowish patch that forms on the sclera, typically at the three- or nine o'clock position adjacent to the cornea. There may be more than one pinguecula present in each eye. A pinguecula completely different from jaundice, which causes a generalized yellowing of the entire sclera. As well, they are differentiated from a pterygium, which grows over the surface of the cornea.

A pinguecula is thought to be caused by exposure to excessive UV light, dust, or wind, and are common in farmers, gardeners, lifeguards, surfers, and construction workers. Most practitioners believe that they do not need to be removed since they do not affect the vision of the patient. However, aside from being unsightly, a pinguecula does tend to swell when irritated, but they return to a stable condition once the irritant has been removed.

## CONVENTIONAL TREATMENT

Currently, there is no medical treatment for a pinguecula because they are not sight-threatening. They are more cosmetically unappealing than dangerous. However, the presence of a pinguecula does indicate that the eye is under environmental stress, and that some action needs to be taken to remedy the situation. In general, the conventional treatment for a pinguecula is to reduce the irritation to the eye. Many doctors simply recommend over-the-counter eye lubricants

## SELF-TREATMENT

Soothing eyewash is the best remedy to quiet a pinguecula that is irritated. Use the herbal remedies below as eyewashes. *Do not* recommend OTC eye drops that are intended to whiten the eye. Council patients to stay out of irritating environments, and wear sunglasses when outdoors for extended periods of time.

| NUTRITIONAL SUPPLEMENTS | | |
|---|---|---|
| **Supplement** | **Directions for Use** | **Comments** |
| Vitamin A | Take 25,000 IU daily. | Good for epithelial cell integrity. |
| Vitamin C | Take 2,000–6,000 mg daily in divided doses. | Protects the eye, and aids tissue healing. |
| Zinc | Take 25 mg daily. | Enhances the immune response. |
| Capsanthin | 40 mg daily | Maintains proper tear film |

| HERBS AND HERBAL SUPPLEMENTS | | |
|---|---|---|
| **Herb** | **Directions for Use** | **Comments** |
| Chamomile | Apply as a hot compress or use as an eyewash. | Soothing for the eye tissues. |
| Eyebright and fennel | Apply as a hot compress or use as an eyewash. | Good for inflammation. |

| HOMEOPATHIC REMEDIES | | |
|---|---|---|
| **Remedy** | **Directions for Use** | **Comments** |
| Apis mellifica 6c | Place 3–4 pellets under the tongue 3–4 times daily. | Relieves swelling around the eyes. |
| Pulsatilla 6c | Place 3–4 pellets under the tongue 3–4 times daily. | Good for eyelids that are stuck together. |
| Ruta graveolens 6c | Place 3–4 pellets under the tongue 3–4 times daily. | Good for hot, red eyes. |
| Sulphur 6c | Place 3–4 pellets under the tongue 3–4 times daily. | Good for red eyelids. |

## RECOMMENDATIONS TO PATIENTS

- Watch your cholesterol level. Some experts feel that a pinguecula might indicate a high blood-cholesterol level. However, no research has as yet been conducted to explore this connection.
- If you believe that you may have a pinguecula, return to the clinic to confirm and allay any fears that your condition is more serious.

# PTERYGIUM

A pterygium has some similarity to a pinguecula, but is shaped differently, is located in a different spot in the eye, and typically has more blood vessels. A pinguecula is a yellowish patch on the white part of the eye. (See *Pinguecula* for a complete discussion.)

A pterygium is a triangular-shaped white area containing a "leash" of blood vessels that seem to feed into the tissue. In fact, the word "pterygium" comes from the Greek word for "wing." While a pinguecula does not interfere with vision and therefore does not need to be removed, a pterygium grows onto the cornea, where it can obscure vision, and therefore should eventually be removed.

Pterygia are usually bilateral located on the nasal side of the cornea but often more prominent on one side. No exact cause for pterygia is known, but the condition does occur more frequently in hot, dusty climates, and it is often seen among surfers (often termed "surfers-eye"), who spend hours in the windy ocean spray and sun.

## CONVENTIONAL TREATMENT

Most eye doctors prefer to leave pterygia alone until they begin to encroach on the line of sight, where they can interfere with vision. Previously, pterygia tended to grow back after being removed. However, the newer procedures are more effective at removing them, and re-growth is now rare. Sometimes a graft of tissue from underneath the inside of the upper eyelid is used to cover the area from the removed tissue. While this is still a complicated procedure, it can be very effective in looking good and feeling good afterward.

| NUTRITIONAL SUPPLEMENTS | | |
|---|---|---|
| **Supplement** | **Directions for Use** | **Comments** |
| Vitamin A | Take 10,000 IU daily. | Good for epithelial cell integrity |
| Vitamin C | Take 2,000–6,000 mg daily in divided doses. | Protects the eye, and aids tissue healing. |
| Zinc | Take 50 mg daily. | Enhances the immune response. |
| Capsanthin | 40 mg daily | Supports the tear film |

| HERBS AND HERBAL SUPPLEMENTS | | |
|---|---|---|
| **Herb** | **Directions for Use** | **Comments** |
| Chamomile | Apply as a hot compress or use as an eyewash. | Soothing for the eye tissues. |
| Eyebright and fennel | Apply as a hot compress or use as an eyewash. | Boost the circulation. |

| HOMEOPATHIC REMEDIES | | |
|---|---|---|
| **Remedy** | **Directions for Use** | **Comments** |
| Acidium Sulfuricum | Place 3-4 pellets under the tongue 3-4 times daily | Resolves pH imbalances |
| Apis mellifica 6c | Place 3–4 pellets under the tongue 3–4 times daily. | Relieves swelling around the eyes. |
| Bellis perrenis | Place 3–4 pellets under the tongue 3–4 times daily. | Helps with healing and capillary weakness |
| Cantharis | Place 3–4 pellets under the tongue 3–4 times daily. | Increases kidney excretion of toxins |
| Lachesis | Place 3–4 pellets under the tongue 3–4 times daily. | Reduces inflammation |
| Ruta graveolens 6c | Place 3–4 pellets under the tongue 3–4 times daily. | Good for hot, red eyes. |
| Sulphur 6c | Place 3–4 pellets under the tongue 3–4 times daily. | Good for red eyelids. |

## RECOMMENDATIONS TO PATIENTS

- Once a pterygium has started to grow, the best thing you can do is to reduce the environmental assault on it.
- Stay out of windy, dusty, sunny, and smoky environments.
- In addition, keep your eyes lubricated and moist.
- Wear good quality sunglasses that block out 100% of UV radiation.

# RETINITIS PIGMENTOSA

Retinitis pigmentosa (RP) is an inherited disease that affects approximately 1 out of every 3,700 people. RP causes deterioration of the retina with progressive loss of sight starting at about the age of ten. The first symptoms are increasing night blindness and difficulty seeing in dim light. Eventually peripheral vision gradually decreases, until the person experiences "tunnel vision" Fortunately, the functional central vision may last until the person is well along in years. However, the loss of peripheral vision will eventually make it impossible for the person to drive or do many mobile tasks.

The retina of these patients will exhibit a classic appearance of "bone spicules", which are actually clumping of pigment, in the periphery. This disease is caused by a mutation in the genes in the photoreceptors, which break down and result in vision loss.

## CONVENTIONAL TREATMENT

The medical community has no treatment for RP. Medical practitioners recommend getting in touch with a low-vision clinic and using the best low-vision aids you can obtain.

However, a breakthrough in tackling retinitis pigmentosa was made by a team of molecular geneticists in New Zealand. The researchers found defects in two genes in the retinal epithelium. They discovered that a number of retinal diseases are caused by genetic mutations in the RPE. The two defective genes give instructions to two proteins that play a vital role in transporting vitamin A to the photoreceptors, which need a continuous supply of the nutrient to function. These researchers believe certain RP cases can be cured by supplementation with raised levels of vitamin A, something that has been suspected for many years, but could not be proven. The mineral zinc most often accomplishes this transport of Vitamin A, thus increased zinc is being considered as a treatment. The drawback of excessive zinc, such as urinary tract issues must be overcome.

Another line of research has centered around "neuroinflammation". Although mutations are the primary cause of RP, research over the past decades has shown that neuroinflammation is an important cause of RP progression. Due to the abnormal activation of immunity, continuous sterile inflammation results in neuron loss and structural destruction. Therapies targeting inflammation have shown their potential to attenuate photoreceptor degeneration in preclinical models. Regardless of variations in genetic background, inflammatory modulation is emerging as an important role in the treatment of RP.

The ancient Egyptians treated "blindness" with ground-up roasted ox liver, a high source of vitamin A. One of the New Zealand researchers conducted much of his practical research in India, in communities where intermarriage and large families are common. This researcher said that it might take generations to prove vitamin A is a preventive cure. But for some known sufferers, vitamin A treatment could be as dramatic as insulin treatment is for diabetics.

Nutritional intervention has also been shown to slow visual field loss associated with retinitis pigmentosa. The National Eye Institute recommends that most adult patients with the common forms of retinitis pigmentosa take a supplement of 15,000 IU of vitamin A daily under the supervision of their eyecare professional. A study published in April 2010 suggests that the addition of 12 mg per day of lutein to this vitamin A regimen can slow the loss of mid-peripheral field sensitivity to a greater degree than vitamin A alone.

For persons with RP who do not respond to vitamin A, another treatment possibility is transplantation of the epithelial layer. This technology, which is already within grasp, may offer a cure to up to one-third of RP sufferers. There are many research studies being conducted but none have proven to be the final answer as of yet.

| NUTRITIONAL SUPPLEMENTS | | |
|---|---|---|
| **Supplement** | **Directions for Use** | **Comments** |
| Vitamin A | Take 75,000 IU daily. | Good for all retinal conditions. *Note:* Use the emulsion form for easier assimilation and greater safety. |
| Essential Fatty Acids | Up to 1500 mg Omega-3 | Supports membrane sensitivity |
| epigallocatechin-3-gallate (EGCG) | 600 mg daily | Anti-inflammatory |
| Lutein | 20 mg daily | Blue light absorption |
| Zeaxanthin | 5 mg daily | Supports macular health |
| Zinc | Up to 40 mg daily | Aids in the transport of Vitamin A |

| HOMEOPATHIC REMEDIES | | |
|---|---|---|
| **Remedy** | **Directions for Use** | **Comments** |
| Nux vomica 6c | Place 3–4 pellets under the tongue 3–4 times daily. | Good for nerve inflammation. |
| Phosphorus 6c | Place 3–4 pellets under the tongue 3–4 times daily. | Supports nerve and vascular integrity. |

## STYE

*See* Hordeolum.

## SUBCONJUNCTIVAL HEMORRHAGE

A subconjunctival hemorrhage is bleeding from a broken blood vessel under the conjunctiva. It is a problem that looks much more serious than it is. A subconjunctival hemorrhage can result from a jarring injury, such as a blow to the head, or from anything that increases the pressure in the delicate blood vessels of the conjunctiva, such as intense coughing, sneezing, vomiting, or pushing during childbirth. The area where the bleeding occurs appears as a bright red patch on the visible portion of the sclera. There is no pain, and vision is not affected.

### CONVENTIONAL TREATMENT

Since the blood will be absorbed and the eye will return to normal within one to three weeks, a subconjunctival hemorrhage does not need to be treated. However, since subconjunctival hemorrhages are often caused by trauma to the eye, it is important to perform a dilated exam to assure that all of the structures of the eye are intact and functioning normally.

### SELF-TREATMENT

If you notice a subconjunctival hemorrhage and it is known when received, have the patient apply cold compresses to the closed eyelid for the first day or two. This will slow any bleeding. For the next day or two, do nothing, then begin to apply warm compresses. This treatment will help the pooled blood to break down more quickly and the condition to resolve. In any case, a subconjunctival hemorrhage will usually disappear on its own in a short time.

| NUTRITIONAL SUPPLEMENTS | | |
|---|---|---|
| **Supplement** | **Directions for Use** | **Comments** |
| Calcium and magnesium | Take 1,000–1,500 mg of a combination supplement daily. | Essential for blood clotting. |
| Vitamin A | Take 5,000 IU daily. | Good for all eye conditions. |
| Vitamin C | Take 3,000 mg daily. | Important for blood clotting. |

| HERBS AND HERBAL SUPPLEMENTS | | |
|---|---|---|
| **Herb** | **Directions for Use** | **Comments** |
| Alfalfa | Take as directed on the label. | A good source of vitamin K. |

| HOMEOPATHIC REMEDIES | | |
|---|---|---|
| **Remedy** | **Directions for Use** | **Comments** |
| Arnica montana 6c | Place 3–4 pellets under the tongue 3–4 times daily. | Good for subconjunctival hemorrhage caused by injury. Reduces hemorrhaging and venous congestion. |
| Sanguinaria 6c | Place 3–4 pellets under the tongue 3–4 times daily. | Improves vasomotor activity, and reduces congestion. |

## RECOMMENDATIONS TO PATIENTS

- As soon as you notice this condition, apply a cold compress (ice) to the closed eyelid. About 20 minutes at a time; a few times a day. After 3 days, start applying a warm compress to the same area.
- If you experience subconjunctival hemorrhages frequently, especially without apparent causes, you should consult your internist.

# PART III
# NUTRITIONAL APPROACHES

# INTRODUCTION

WHILE WE ARE EYE CARE PROVIDERS, WE SHOULD BE AWARE OF VARIOUS modalities that cover all health aspects of the human condition. Western medicine certainly has its benefits and requirements but there is a distinction between a disease and "dis-ease". That is more than just a play on words. It has been said that the American medical system is not "healthcare" but more "disease management". In the medical field, it is called "functional medicine", whereby the doctor takes a more holistic approach to resolving any health issues. This includes diet, exercise, smoking, herbal treatments, homeopathy, acupuncture, and other modalities.

Here we will list some of these "alternatives" to the basic medical model of health. While this is different that CAM (Complementary and Alternative Medicine), there are some similarities. Functional medicine doesn't disapprove of required medical management but also looks to optimal health and lifestyle to achieve a long- and healthy- life. As an old Ayurvedic saying goes, "When diet is wrong, medicine is of no use; when diet is correct, medicine is of no need".

# A DIET FOR HEALTHY EYES

For most people, the word *diet* is synonymous with starvation, restriction and a miserable lifestyle. In other words, it's a "four-letter word". The fact that nutritional advice is often confusing and frustrating only compounds its negativity. One day, a certain food or supplement is good for us; the next day, it is not. Nevertheless, the truth remains that the foods we eat play a major role in all aspects of overall health, as well as eye health.

As humans, we are the result of many years of evolution; a combination of natural selection and our genetic inheritance. Research has shown that our genes have changed very little in the last 40,000 years. We have the same genetic makeup as our primitive hunter-gatherer ancestors from 10,000 years ago. What we know today is that the foods we eat are chemical triggers that can turn our genetic expression on and off.

Proper nutrition for vision and eye health, and health in general, requires that we eat foods that are "gene friendly." This means eating a diet of foods that contribute to turning the health-promoting genes on and turning the disease-promoting genes off.

Our stone-age ancestors ate a wide variety of wild plant and animal foods so that their diets consisted of healthy meats and animal organs, fish, shellfish, eggs, fruits, nuts, seeds, berries and complex carbohydrates in the form of wild plants, roots, and vegetables.

This "gene-friendly" diet provided four basic things:

1. The right balance of saturated and unsaturated fats for cell membranes and nerve function;
2. Complex carbohydrates for fiber and the maintenance of stable blood-glucose and insulin levels;
3. High quality plant and animal protein for enzymes, muscles and other body tissue;
4. An abundance of essential vitamins, minerals and phytochemicals to act as antioxidants and enzyme system catalysts.

Notice that each of these categories call for a *balance* of nutrients. Our modern Western diet of processed foods with their high levels of refined grains, modern vegetable oils, sugar, salt and chemical additives, and low in important nutrients, is turning on genes that promote inflammation and chronic disease. When it affects the genes that control the eye, it can lead to the vision-threatening conditions of macular degeneration, cataracts, myopia, and diabetic and hypertensive retinopathy. This is borne out when we call our "Standard American Diet" the "SAD" diet!

## THE IDEAL HUMAN DIET FOR GOOD VISION

While there is really not any "perfect' diet for every person, there are some general concepts that we know are the right things to do. For one, we need the right balance of saturated and unsaturated fats for cell membranes and nerve function. In numerous studies on the effects of dietary fat on health, the results have shown that it is not the total fat content that is a concern, but the balance of fats. Animal fats and oils were a very important part of primitive people's diets, so much so that they were celebrated in their myths and legends. Nearly all hunted and gathered foods were perceived to be enhanced by adding oil. We should not be afraid of fat in our diet. We don't get fat from eating fat! Fats from wild animals and fish, nuts and seeds eaten in moderate amounts, provide a good source of energy and the right balance of building materials for healthy cells and nerves.

Our "SAD" Western diet is out of balance with too much saturated fat and too much grain-based polyunsaturated omega-6 fats found in modern processed vegetable oils and our grain-fed cattle which contribute to inflammation. Less saturated fat and more monounsaturated and omega-3 fats from green plants, grass-fed animals and wild caught fish can help restore the dietary balance of fats to which we are genetically adapted, thus reducing inflammation.

Complex carbohydrates are needed for fiber and the maintenance of stable blood-glucose and insulin levels. However, our Western diet is overloaded with refined grains, starches and sugars. These foods are digested and absorbed rapidly causing blood sugar and insulin levels to rise quickly. These rapid elevations in sugar and insulin lead to almost as rapid a decline in sugar and insulin in the blood, leading to chronically unstable blood sugar levels and disease processes such as diabetes. (See Figures 1 through 6.)

The wild green plants (a good source of omega-3 fats) and the various fruits and non-starchy vegetables cause only a limited rise in blood sugar while providing needed fiber for intestinal health. The carbohydrate content of fruits and vegetables is low compared to cereal grains, and contain far more vitamins and minerals.

Cereal grains contain natural chemical substances called "phytates" that can inhibit the absorption of vitamins and minerals. Unless grains are properly prepared by soaking, sprouting or fermenting to neutralize the phytates and other toxins, these substances can contribute to nutrient deficiencies. Many native people used soaking and fermenting as food preservation techniques and they benefited from the enhanced nutritional properties that resulted since the proteins, vitamins and minerals could be absorbed more easily from these foods. Today's refined cereal grain foods are fortified with minerals and synthetic vitamins in part to offset the anti-nutrient effects of phytates and other such substances.

High quality plant and animal protein are needed for enzymes, muscles and other body tissue. Protein is essential for our body to build muscle and other tissues. Protein also satisfies hunger more than fat and carbohydrates. However, too much protein can lead to an excess of nitrogen in the body and make us ill, and should be eaten with complex carbohydrates from fresh fruits and vegetables and with moderate well-balanced amounts of fats and oils. Protein does not interfere with blood-sugar and insulin levels. It also helps with weight loss since it stimulates our metabolism more than fats or carbohydrates.

An abundance of essential vitamins, minerals and phytochemicals to act as antioxidants and enzyme system catalysts are critical. Essential phytochemicals such as carotenoids, bioflavonoids and polyphenols are found in the skins and pulp of berries and other colorful plant foods. Their antioxidant and anti-inflammatory properties are vital for good vision and eye health.

An ideal diet contains a variety of free-range protein (including fish, poultry and beef) making up, on average, about half of their food energy. Various wild plants provide the remaining half of their food calories.

The dietary fat intake should range from 30 to 60 percent of the total calories with a moderate amount of fat calories from polyunsaturated fatty acids found naturally in meats, fish, nuts, seeds and other plants. The balance of fat calories should come from high amounts of monounsaturated fatty acids and moderate amounts of saturated fatty acids. An ideal diet should contain a ratio of omega-6 to omega-3 essential fatty acids of about 4 to 1. (Our Western dietary ratio is estimated to be nearly 30 to 1.)

Regarding meat, it's important to be mindful of what type of fat and meat one is consuming. Meat is acidifying to the body. Cancer cells thrive in an acidic environment (which is why sugars are also so bad for decreasing immunity and promoting cancer). Additionally, there is a huge difference between organic, free-range, grass-fed animals versus commercially raised animals with respect to chemicals, pesticides and hormones which accumulate in the animals' fat. Just like us, stressed animals produce excessive cortisol which stays in the tissues.

Grains, seeds and nuts ideally should be soaked and sprouted to reduce the "anti-nutrients" and help with digestion. So, in moderation they can be part of a healthy diet. Many nutritionists recommend a 55%

raw, organic vegetable diet. Protein, good fats and complex carbohydrates should be eaten in moderation. The key is to be 80% alkaline (raw vegetables, high mineral content). Too much protein can leach the body of calcium (bi-products of protein metabolism include ammonia). If you cannot get enough energy from glucose (coming from carbohydrates) then the body will start to burn its own fat leading to the release of ketones which can lead to ketoacidosis which can damage liver and kidney. More on that in the section on the Keto Diet below.

## VARIOUS DIET PROGRAMS

So, why should eyecare professionals be concerned with patients' diets? Consider that there are over 60 studies that link excessive weight to chronic eye disease. This indicates a connection that we need to be concerned with and make appropriate referrals to nutrition practitioners. We will discuss the "eye-gut" connection later in this section. When working together, eyecare and nutrition practitioners can help guide patients to make the right choices in their food plan that will benefit not only their eyes but their life- and health-span as well. The following diet programs are listed to give you an overall view of the concepts that they support. Again, while no one program is perfect for everyone, co-managing patients with a qualified nutritionist will allow you to contribute to your patients' overall health.

### ATKINS DIET

The Atkins diet, which has been around since the 1960s, has gained worldwide attention as a way to eat a lot of food, not be hungry and still lose weight. The Atkins Diet works on the theory that carbohydrates cause you to gain weight, and by eliminating or strictly limiting carbohydrates, it is possible to eat a lot of protein and fat while your weight decreases. When you do not consume carbohydrates, your body is forced to convert fat stores into carbohydrates, which is an inefficient process. So, your body uses its fat stores at a faster rate and you lose weight.

This theory seems beneficial to dieters, especially for overweight diabetes patients who have trouble metabolizing carbohydrates due to insulin problems. With the Atkins system, diabetes and pre-diabetes patients are encouraged to eat as few as 20 grams of carbohydrate a day for successful diabetes weight loss. There is no limitation on protein and fat (both saturated and unsaturated) consumption.

The Atkins diet has generated its share of criticism. First, it recommends eating greater amounts of animal protein and fat, and these foods cause people to lose a lot of water from their bodies. In turn, this puts extra strain on the kidneys, which are usually already weakened in people with diabetes. While a traditional approach to weight loss focuses on limiting refined sugars and foods which release sugars, this type of diet may contain an unhealthful amount of fat and protein. Due to this heavy consumption of high saturated fat red meat, the Atkins diet is also thought to increase the chance for heart disease. Finally, the Atkins diet can lead to dangerously low blood sugar levels (hypoglycemia). For a person with diabetes, extremely low blood sugar can lead to a coma. Most experts agree that using the Atkins diet for diabetes can be risky and should not be attempted without medical supervision.

## THE KETOGENIC DIET

Ketogenic diets are very high in fat and very low in carbohydrates and protein. This concept is similar to the Adkin's diet. In fact, some of the latest research shows that a modified Atkins diet is just as good as the ketogenic diet. The classic ketogenic diet uses a ratio of 4:1:1 for fat, carbohydrate, and protein. Some people consider ketogenic diets to be extremely difficult and unappetizing, whereas low-carb dieters tend to find such discouragement silly.

The keto diet requires a major commitment since your body will not go into ketosis immediately. It may take several weeks to achieve the ketosis you need to lose accumulated fat. Thus, it's easy to get frustrated and more difficult to stick to the diet. Most authorities suggest a keto diet as an "entry point" to losing weight, whereby you stick to the diet for a few weeks, then gradually increase your carbs to a "normal" level again.

## THE MEDITERRANEAN DIET

Based on food patterns typical of Crete, much of the rest of Greece and southern Italy in the early 1960s, the Mediterranean diet, in addition to regular physical activity, emphasizes abundant plant foods, fresh fruit as the typical daily dessert, olive oil as the principal source of fat, dairy products (principally cheese and yogurt), and fish and poultry consumed in low to moderate amounts, zero to four eggs consumed weekly, red meat consumed in low amounts, and wine consumed in low to moderate amounts. Total fat in this diet is 25-35 percent of calories, with saturated fat at 8 percent or less of calories.

Studies have shown that people with type 2 diabetes on a Mediterranean diet were better able to manage their disease without diabetes medications than those who ate a low-fat diet with no more than 30 percent of calories from fat (less than 10 percent coming from saturated fat choices). After four years, researchers found that 44 percent of people on the Mediterranean diet ended up requiring diabetes medications to control their blood sugars compared with 70 percent of those who followed the low-fat diet.

Dietary factors are only part of the reason for the health benefits enjoyed by certain Mediterranean cultures. A healthy lifestyle, notably a physically active lifestyle or labor is also beneficial. Environment may also be involved. For the population of a whole country or a region, the influence of genetics is rather minimal, because it was shown that the slowly changing habits of Mediterranean populations, from a healthy active lifestyle and Mediterranean diet to a not so healthy, less physically active lifestyle and a diet influenced by the Western pattern diet, significantly increases risk of heart disease. There is an inverse association between adherence to the Mediterranean diet and the incidence of fatal and non-fatal heart disease in initially healthy middle-aged adults in the Mediterranean region.

## THE PALEO DIET

The Paleolithic, or Paleo diet is based on the premise that modern humans are genetically adapted to the diet of their Paleolithic ancestors and that human genetics have scarcely changed since the dawn of agriculture. Therefore, that an ideal diet for human health and well-being is one that resembles this ancestral diet. For almost all of our evolutionary history, humans and human ancestors survived on hunter-gatherer diets.

Proponents of this diet argue that modern human populations subsisting on traditional diets allegedly similar to those of Paleolithic hunter-gatherers are largely free of diseases of affluence. Supporters point to several potentially therapeutic nutritional characteristics of pre-agricultural diets. This included lean meats, seafood, vegetables, fruits and nuts, and it is lower in cereals and dairy products. It was also higher in unsaturated fatty acids, dietary cholesterol and several vitamins. It is lower in total energy, energy density, carbohydrate, dietary glycemic load (GL), glycemic index (GI), saturated fatty acids and calcium. Studies have concluded that a Paleolithic diet improved glycemic control and several cardiovascular risk factors as compared to a diabetes diet. The Paleolithic diet produces lower A1c, triglycerides and diastolic blood pressure, as well as lower weight, body mass index (BMI), waist circumference and higher HDL (good) cholesterol.

Because they ate wild game, including organ meats and brains, our Paleolithic ancestors consumed higher amounts of omega-3 fatty acids and lower amounts of omega-6. They also had high vitamin D levels as a result of the sun exposure they received from living outside. Both of these nutrients have powerful health benefits. To maintain adequate omega-3 intake and vitamin D levels, most modern humans will need to supplement with fish or krill oil, and vitamin D. Many people take cod liver oil because it contains both omega-3 and vitamin D; however, it also contains preformed vitamin A that antagonizes the action of vitamin D. Thus, if you do recommend cod-liver oil, it should be taken only in small doses (½ teaspoon daily).

There are many misconceptions regarding this diet. Here are several myths and the truth for each:

- *You Need to Live Like a Caveman*—You don't have to mimic the Paleolithic lifestyle. There is no need to live in caves. Eating whole, unprocessed foods and natural foods is what the diet promotes.
- *It's an Unbalanced and Meat-only Diet*—A typical paleo meal consists of a small portion of meat with lots of veggies, fruit and nuts. By volume, Paleo dieters eat a lot more plant food by volume.
- *Paleo is a Fad*—The Paleo lifestyle goes all the way back to Paleolithic times. The fundamental premise of the diet is to eat the foods our bodies were designed to eat. This only proves that Paleo is not a short-lived fad.
- *It's Expensive*—You don't necessarily need to have only prime cuts of meat. A study found that the Paleo Diet was feasible even using the USDA's Thrifty Food Plan.
- *You Don't Get Enough Calcium*—The reduction of dairy causes alarm for some people but the truth is, you can get this mineral from eating green vegetables.
- *No More Carbs*—Actually, there are still a healthy amount of carbs. The Paleo Diet has just fewer carbs than the current recommendations, which many in the nutrition world are now agreeing are too high. The suggested amount of carbs for the average American by the CDC is 130 mg daily.
- *You Starve from Small Portions*—The truth is that you don't need to count calories. People are challenged to eat as much healthy vegetables, fruit and lean meat as they want and overeat. They can't do it!
- *Goodbye Normal Food*—Unlike other strict diets, Paleo lets you have a variety of food. The 85 percent rule even lets you have your favorite snack once a week. It's about diversifying your diet.

- *Your Lifespan Shortens*—Life back then was pretty dangerous because of the lack of sanitation, dangers from wild animals and the surroundings. A broken leg was a death sentence. Few lived to old-age but those who did, lived longer. Also, they didn't suffer from obesity, diabetes or other diseases that have proliferated in our time.

## RAW FOOD DIET

An extension of the vegetarian diet is a raw food diet. A raw vegan diet consists of unprocessed, raw plant foods that have not been heated above 40 °C (104 °F). Raw vegans believe that foods cooked above this temperature have lost much of their nutritional value and are less healthful or even harmful to the body. Advocates argue that raw or living foods have natural enzymes, which are critical in building proteins and rebuilding the body, and that heating these foods kills the natural enzymes and can leave toxins behind. However, critics point out those enzymes, as with other proteins consumed in the diet, are denatured and eventually lysed by the digestive process rendering them non-functional. Typical foods included in raw food diets are fruits, vegetables, nuts, seeds and sprouted grains and legumes.

Raw foodists believe that raw foods are the ideal food for human consumption, and the basis of a raw food lifestyle. Irritants or stimulants like coffee, alcohol, and tobacco are taboo. Also heated fats and proteins like fried oils and roasted nuts are to be avoided, as they are deemed to be carcinogenic.

Wild foods followed by organic whole foods are more nutritious than conventionally domesticated foods or industrially produced foods. The theory is that cooked foods contain harmful toxins, which can cause chronic disease and other problems. Heating oils and fats can produce trace amounts of trans fats. Cooking foods produces advanced glycation end products (AGEs), which is apparent by the "browning" of meat and other cooked foods. They claim that this same effect occurs in the blood vessels when eating cooked food.

Among raw vegans there are some subgroups such as fruitarians, juicearians, or sproutarians. Fruitarians eat primarily or exclusively fruits, berries, seeds, and nuts. Juicearians process their raw plant foods into juice. Sproutarians adhere to a diet consisting mainly of sprouted seeds.

As a side note for lutein and zeaxanthin consumption in food: these fat-soluble molecules are bound to chlorophyll in green vegetables. If ingested raw, they are less bioavailable than if they are cooked or steamed. For maximum absorption for eye health, spinach and kale (and the like) are best taken cooked. On a practical note, one might suggest alternating consumption between the two options.

## VEGETARIAN DIET

Minimizing fat intake and reducing body fat help insulin to be more effective. Newer recommendations drastically reduce the suggested intake levels of meats, high-fat dairy products and oils. At the same time, this theory increases quantities of grains, legumes, fruits and vegetables. One study found that 21 of 23 patients on oral medications and 13 of 17 patients on insulin were able to get off of their medications after 26 days on a near-vegetarian diet and exercise program. Please note that ALL dietary weight loss programs always add *exercise* to the protocol.

According to the vegetarian model, eating soy foods can lower cholesterol, decrease blood glucose levels and improve glucose tolerance in people with diabetes. Researchers identified the molecular pathway that allows foods rich in soy bioactive compounds, isoflavones, to lower diabetes and heart disease risk. Researchers also found that the isoflavones daidzein and equol enhanced adipocyte differentiation, or the formation of fat cells, through activation of a key transcription regulator, the same receptor that mediates the insulin-sensitizing effects of anti-diabetes drugs. Thus, daidzein and equol seem to work in a similar manner as anti-diabetic drugs currently in the market. Soy isoflavones may exert anti-diabetic effects by targeting fat cell-specific factors and the downstream signaling molecules that are important for glucose uptake and thus insulin sensitivity.

## THE MYOPIA DIET

While you will likely not see this diet listed in any food or nutritional support books or articles, this is a diet that was developed by the author to address the role of diet on the development and progression of myopia. This information was also covered in the section on Myopia.

Over the past 30+ years, evidence has shown that the consumption of a Westernized diet promotes the development of both acute and chronic hyperinsulinemia, which has also been termed "pre-diabetes". Numerous studies have demonstrated that the addition of sucrose in the diet of both normal and hyperinsulinemia subjects causes an increase in postprandial insulin levels. There is evidence that insulin has direct ocular growth promoting effects as well as indirect effects via the induction of insulin like growth factors leading to decreased insulin-like growth factor binding protein (IGFBP), also implicated in ocular growth.

Collectively, these studies show that increasing consumption of high levels of refined carbohydrates, especially those considered high caloric foods, is particularly responsible for the worsening of glycemic control, and therefore insulin resistance and compensatory hyperinsulinemia

The metabolic reactions that accompany hyperinsulinemia are complex and have profound effects on growth and development, including within the eye. Post-prandial levels of insulin are produced by the pancreas, while the liver secretes insulin-like growth factor-1 (IGF-1) as well as the IGFBP-1, which controls the action of IGF-1. Hyperinsulinemia suppresses the secretion of IGFBP-1 from the liver, which in turn increases free IGF-1 in the serum.10 Increased circulating levels of free IGF-1 is a potent stimulator of growth in all tissue. See the flowchart at the end of this chapter

Retinoic acid, which is required for growth and development, is a metabolite of vitamin A that mediates the functions of the vitamin. The all-trans-retinoic acid (ATRA) form is essential in growth of higher animals. During early embryonic development, ATRA helps determine the orientation of the posterior portion of the embryo. In the sclera, ATRA inhibits glycosaminoglycan synthesis, thereby thinning the sclera and promoting axial elongation.

Many nutrients are required for proper growth and development. A balance of 13 essential vitamins and 15 essential minerals is critical for proper utilization. Some of these nutrients have been associated with the development of myopia, specifically vitamin A (as discussed above), vitamin B2 and vitamin C.

Vitamin B2 (riboflavin) is involved in energy metabolism, cell respiration, antibody production, growth and development and are essential for the metabolism of carbohydrates, protein and fats. Additionally, riboflavin is involved in the metabolism of niacin, vitamin B6, and folate. Riboflavin is used in the currently established process of collagen crosslinking, which is an effective method for halting the progression of keratectasia in patients with keratoconus. Given the effects of UVA on collagen, one could postulate an internal interaction of riboflavin and UVA radiation with time spent outdoors.

One study showed that oral administration of riboflavin with whole body UVA irradiation could increase the strength and stiffness of the sclera by altering biochemical and biomechanical properties. Another study showed that violet light (VL, 360-400 nm wavelength) suppresses myopia progression, with VL transmitting contact lenses suppressing myopia progression most. The results suggested that VL is one of the important outdoor environmental factors for myopia control. Since VL is apt to be excluded from our modern society due to the excessive UV protection, VL exposure can be a preventive strategy against myopia progression.

Vitamin C is essential for collagen production in the body by serving as a co-factor for two enzymes that are responsible for stabilizing collagen molecules. Vitamin C deficiency leads to impaired collagen synthesis. Vitamin C is water-soluble and flushes out of the body in 2-3 hours, so a single daily dose is not very effective.

Vitamin D has been studied in several trials because of its association to sunlight. Low serum vitamin D is associated with axial length and risk of myopia in young children. However, this effect has not been born out in studies. Yet studies have confirmed that about 90 minutes of outdoor activity per day can be beneficial in early myopia progression. However, it has been shown that 90-120 minutes of outdoor time is effective in preventing myopia. This is most likely due to dopamine levels since bright light stimulates dopamine release in the retina.

Foods that can contribute to collagen structure include bone broth, gelatin, eggs (white), citrus, tomatoes, broccoli, avocados, leafy greens, nuts and mushrooms.

Given the unprecedented rise in myopia in people of Asian and Chinese descent, it is important to review possible trends in their dietary habits. It is documented that this demographic tends to be more insulin resistant than people of European descent. Reviewing the demographics of diabetes world-wide, it should be noted that over half of the world's diabetes population is centered in Western Pacific and Southeast Asian regions. (see Fig. 3) It is possible that the higher rates of myopia in Asian populations may in part be due to their increased genetic susceptibility to insulin resistance. It is important to note that white rice, which has a glycemic load of 33 (anything over 20 is considered high), is a staple of the diet in Asia.

It is possible that the etiology of juvenile onset myopia does not have a single cause but might be a result of a "perfect storm" of a number of factors. It has been established that newborns typically exhibit low hyperopia. When taking in a westernized diet that includes highly refined grains and carbohydrates, they could likely tend toward development of hyperinsulinemia. The growth pattern of the sclera thins and continues to elongate due to the excessive carbohydrate influences, combined with a lack of outdoor lighting and an increase of near point tasks (especially the digital display variety). This depleted nutrition pattern might continue with a vitamin B2 deficiency and intraocular pressure increases with the excessive accommodation leading to continued scleral elongation and subsequent myopia. Real world human studies would be required to confirm how these interactions might lead to the current state of myopia development.

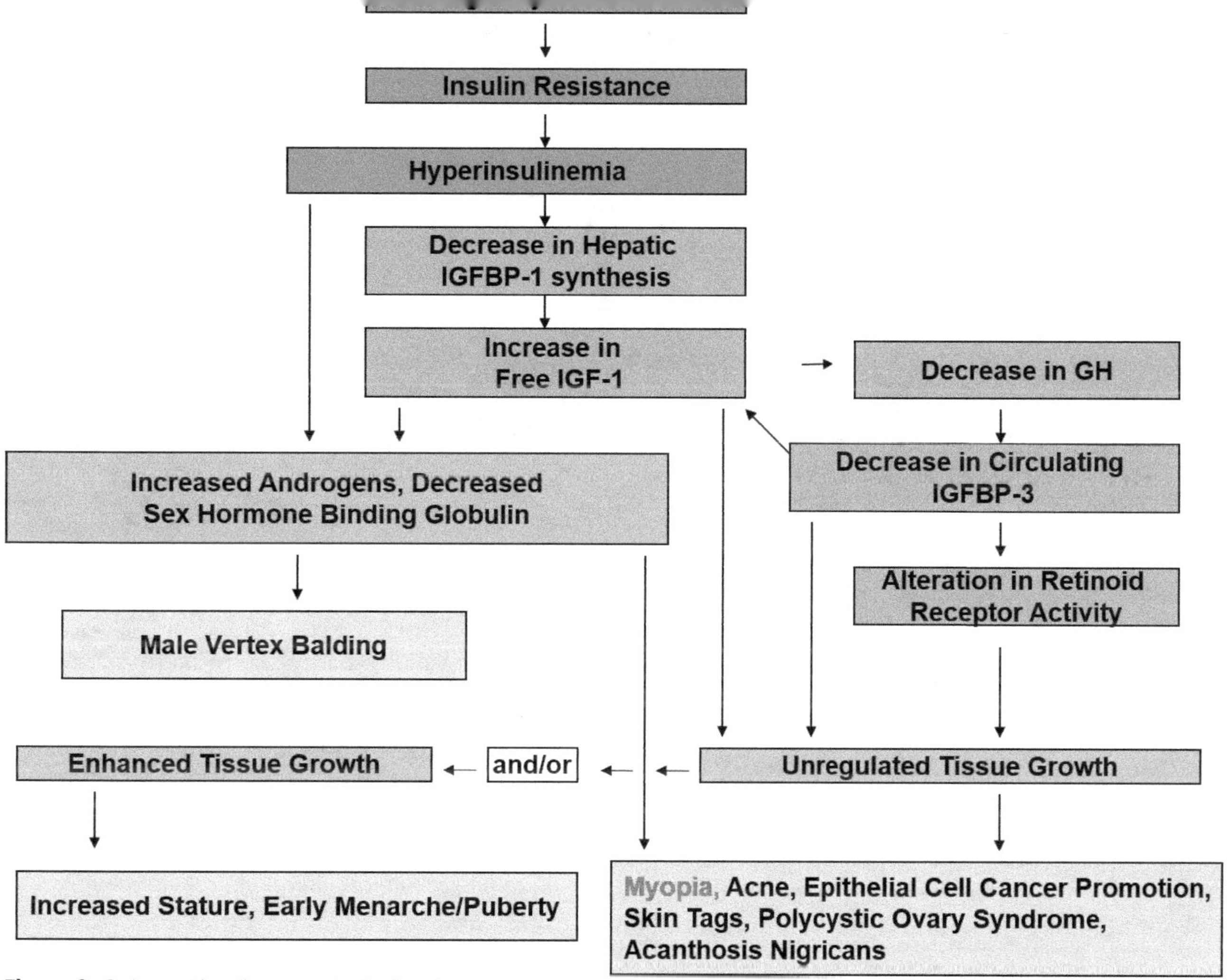


**Figure 2.** Schematic diagram depicting how compensatory hyperinsulinaemia facilitates unregulated scleral tissue growth via increases in IGF-1 and attenuation of the retinoic acid signal. COURTESY LOREN CORDAIN, PHD

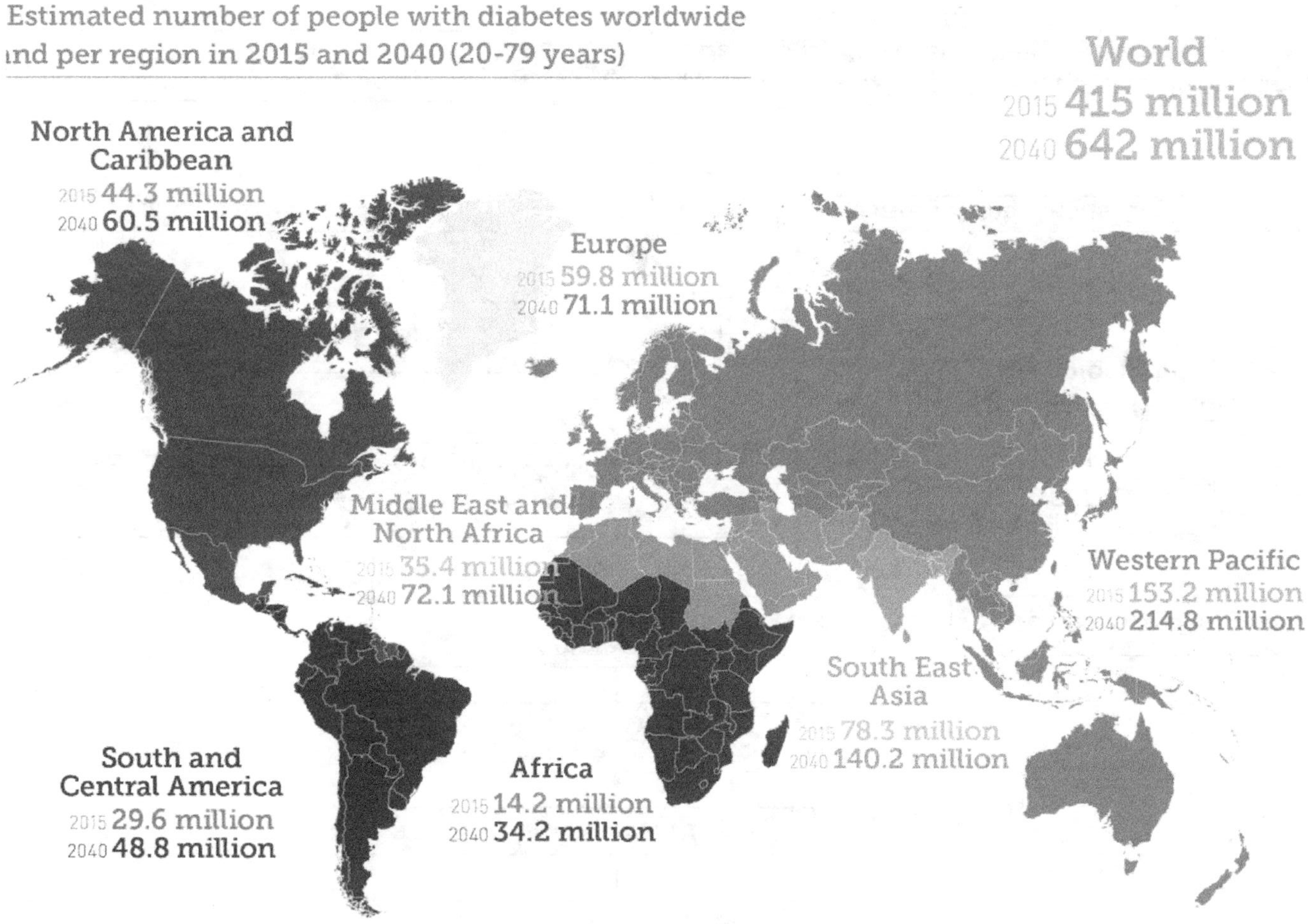


**Figure 3.** Number of people with diabetes worldwide as estimated. COURTESY OF THE INTERNATIONAL DIABETES FEDERATION

## COMPARISON OF DIETS

| Nutrients | Traditional | Paleolithic | Low-Carb | Low-Fat Because oxidative stress contributes Vegetarian |
|---|---|---|---|---|
| Common Name | Mediterranean | Hunter-Gatherer | Atkins-type | Ornish-type |
| Protein | Moderate (16-23%) | High (19-35%) | Moderate (18-23%) | Low (<15%) |
| Carbohydrates | Moderate (50%) | Moderate (22-40%) | Low (4-26%) | High (80%) |
| Total Fat | Moderate (30%) | Moderate (28-47%) | High (51-78%) | Low (<10%) |
| Saturated Fat | Low | Moderate | High | Low |
| Monounsaturated Fat | High | High | Moderate | Low |
| Polyunsaturated Fat | Moderate | Moderate | Moderate | Low |
| Omega-3 Fat | High | High | Low | Low |
| Total Fiber | High | High | Low | High |
| Fruits/Veggies | High | High | Low | High |
| Nuts and Seeds | Moderate | Moderate | Low | Low |
| Salt | Moderate | Low | High | Low |
| Refined Sugars | Low | Low | Low | Low |
| Glycemic Load | Low | Low | Low | High |

## Fats

Speaking of fat, you may be confused about fat and its possible negative impacts on health. Controversy regarding this subject exists even among qualified healthcare professionals. It is unfortunate that we relate fat to "gaining excess weight". We do not get fat from eating fat! In fact, all forms of fat are not created equal. The key word here is "created", as some saturated fats occur naturally, while others are artificially created, such as the saturated fat that comes from the process of hydrogenation. Hydrogenation manipulates vegetable and seed oils by adding hydrogen atoms while heating these substances. This act produces thickened oil that benefits the shelf life of processed foods and gives these edibles a firmer texture.

The medical and scientific communities are now fairly united in the opinion that hydrogenated vegetable and seed oils should be avoided. The artificial fats creased by hydrogenation are called trans fats. There is no controversy regarding the health dangers of these artificial compounds any longer. They have now been banned in food products in the US. However, if you look at a food label that says, "no trans fats", be sure to see if there are hydrogenated (or partially hydrogenated) oils in the product. Companies are allowed to include up to 500 mg of hydrogenated oils in a product and still claim it as "zero" on the label.

# THE GLYCEMIC INDEX (GI)

THE GLYCEMIC INDEX (GI) DESCRIBES HOW CARBOHYDRATE-CONTAINING food affects blood glucose levels. When we eat carbohydrates, our body breaks them down to produce glucose.

For glucose to move from the blood into the body's cells, it needs insulin, which along with glucagon (stimulated through protein intake) plays a key role in determining whether our body burns fat or carbohydrates for energy. The pancreas produces both insulin and glucagon. Whenever glucose is present in the blood, insulin is stimulated; whenever protein is present, glucagon is stimulated. If the insulin is insufficient, however, glucose levels rise. A high level of insulin forces the body to burn carbohydrate rather than fat, which allows fat to accumulate in the body. Therefore, if we control the rate of glucose our body absorbs, we will also control the amount of insulin secreted. This is where the GI comes into play.

The GI is a ranking of carbohydrates on a scale from 0 to 100 according to the extent to which they raise blood sugar levels after eating. Foods and drinks with a high GI (over 55), such as fruit juices, sugary sweets, etc., are those that the body rapidly digests and absorbs and result in an excess of insulin in the bloodstream. Controlling the glucose levels of these foods and drinks allows for control over food-driven insulin stimulation and reactive hypoglycaemia.

Low-GI foods (under 55), by virtue of their slow digestion and absorption, produce a more gradual rise in blood sugar and insulin levels, allowing the body to utilize the glucose formed from the breakdown of complex carbohydrates, instead of storing it in a fat cell as glycogen. When

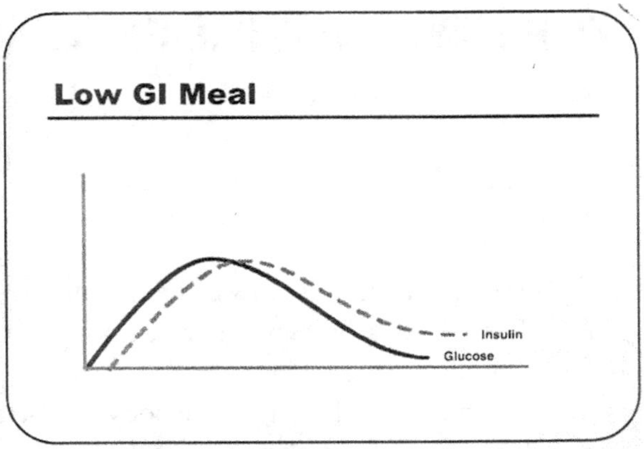


**Figure 4.** For low-glycemic meals, notice the close approximation of the glucose and insulin levels.

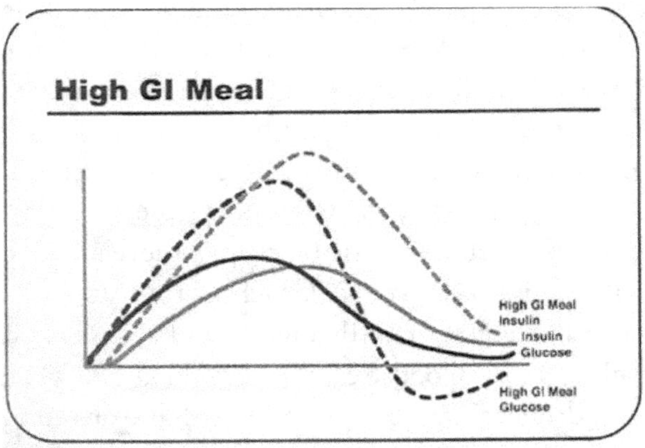


**Figure 5.** Note the large difference between glucose levels and insulin levels in the High GI meal. This results in large amounts of free insulin in the serum which is toxic to blood vessels.

excessive amounts of fat are stored, they enlarge the fat cells in adipose tissue and increase the risk of chronic disease, such as cancer, diabetes, and others. As a result, low-GI foods have proven benefits for health.

While the GI is an important concept, there is also the glycemic load (GL), which is a ranking system for carbohydrate content in food *portions* based on their GI and the portion size.

The usefulness of glycemic load is based on the idea that a high glycemic index food consumed in small quantities would give the same effect as larger quantities of a low glycemic index food on blood sugar. For example, white rice is somewhat high GI, so eating 50 g of white rice at one sitting would give a particular glucose curve in the blood, while 25 g would give the same curve but half the height. Since the peak height is probably the most important parameter, multiplying the amount of carbohydrates in a food serving by the glycemic index gives an idea of how much effect an actual portion of food has on blood sugar level.

Visit www.glycemicindex.com for the index and database. See figure below for various foods.

| Glycemic Index and Glycemic Load for Common Foods | | | | |
|---|---|---|---|---|
| **Food** | **GI** | **Serving Size** | **Net Carbs** | **GL** |
| Peanuts | 14 | 4 oz | 15 | 2 |
| Bean Sprouts | 25 | 1 oz | 4 | 1 |
| Grapefruit | 25 | ½ large | 11 | 3 |
| Pizza | 30 | 2 slices | 42 | 13 |
| Lowfat yogurt | 33 | 1 cup | 47 | 16 |
| Apples | 38 | 1 medium | 16 | 6 |
| Spaghetti | 42 | 1 cup | 38 | 16 |
| Carrots | 47 | 1 large | 5 | 2 |
| Oranges | 48 | 1 medium | 12 | 6 |
| Banana | 52 | 1 large | 27 | 14 |
| Potato Chips | 54 | 4 oz | 55 | 30 |
| Snickers Bar | 55 | 1 bar | 64 | 35 |
| Brown Rice | 55 | 1 cup | 42 | 23 |
| Honey | 55 | 1 tbsp | 17 | 9 |
| Oatmeal | 58 | 1 cup | 21 | 12 |
| Ice cream | 61 | 1 cup | 16 | 10 |
| Macaroni & Cheese | 64 | 1 serving | 47 | 30 |
| Raisins | 64 | 1 small box | 32 | 20 |
| White Rice | 64 | 1 cup | 52 | 33 |
| Sugar (Sucrose) | 68 | 1 tbsp | 12 | 8 |
| White Bread | 70 | 1 slice | 14 | 10 |
| Watermelon | 72 | 1 cup | 11 | 8 |
| Popcorn | 72 | 2 cups | 10 | 7 |
| Baked Potato | 85 | 1 medium | 33 | 28 |
| Glucose | 100 | (50 g) | 50 | 50 |

**Figure 6.** Glycemic Index and Glycemic Load of common foods.

The total glycemic load is the (glycemic index × carb content)/100 of each food. A glycemic load of 20 or higher is considered high.

# NUTRITION FOR THE DIABETIC PATIENT

Diabetes has been diagnosed in over 38.4 million Americans (or 11.6 percent of the population), and 97.6 million more have been diagnosed with pre-diabetes. This disease costs our healthcare system over $412.9 billion per year. New cases of diabetes are more prevalent in the age group from 40 to 59—an increasing trend. (See Figure 3.) Diabetes is the seventh leading cause of death and the leading cause of blindness in adults aged 20 to 74 years. Diabetic retinopathy causes 12,000 to 24,000 new cases of blindness each year. Overall, the risk for death among people with diabetes is about twice that of people without diabetes within similar age groups.

Diabetes poses a major public health challenge because it increases the risk of both large and small blood vessel diseases. Diabetes epidemic has been fueled by increasing rates of overweight and obesity, leading to the term "diabesity", yet surveys showed that a majority of such patients have had no substantive discussions with their physicians about diet and exercise, even those who have been given a diabetes diagnosis. Educating patients about nutrition is of paramount importance since caloric intake and quality determine energy homeostasis and hyperglycemia drives virtually all of the vascular complications of diabetes via distinct pathways moderated by mitochondrial overproduction of reaction oxygen species (ROS). The act of metabolism itself generates ROS. Nutritional counseling also must be considered in light of GI disturbances manifest as diabetic autonomic neuropathy and autoimmune and enteropathy (celiac disease).

As primary eye care providers, we focus time and energy on how to treat the ocular complications associated with diabetes. However, we can do a lot within our scope of practice to prevent type 2 diabetes from ever developing. We need to concentrate on lifestyle modification, including proper dietary strategies and exercise concepts. Here are some tips on how to address some of these with your patients.

## DISCUSSING DIET

There are many concepts of the "proper" diet for any weight control issue, including diabetes prevention. Depending on the severity and length of time the condition has existed, varying amounts of proteins, fats, fiber and carbohydrates are recommended.

The American Diabetes Association recommends a diet consisting of:

- Total fat intake that equals 25 to 35 percent of total calories.
- Saturated fat, less than 7 percent of total calories.
- A total cholesterol intake under 200 mg/d (low-density lipoprotein < 100; high-density lipoprotein > 40).
- Carbohydrate intake equal to about 50 to 60 percent of total calories.
- Fiber between 20gm/d to 30gm/d.

However, many healthcare practitioners find this a poor diet due to the high carbohydrate allowance, since carbohydrate processing is one of the main concerns for a patient with diabetes. Glucose is the body's primary energy source, fueling the activities of nearly every cell in the body.

The availability and storage of blood glucose is tightly controlled by a process called glucose homeostasis, which involves insulin. Insulin is produced by the beta cells of the pancreas in response to changes in blood sugar, and works to maintain blood glucose levels within an optimal range, or homeostasis. Overeating, physical inactivity, and aging result in increased pro-inflammatory cytokine production. The over-production of pro-inflammatory cytokines may represent a triggering factor in the origin of heart, blood sugar, and other metabolic concerns. Thus, reducing carbohydrates reduces the strain on the pancreas to produce more insulin.

And don't forget, a simple "common sense" diet can accomplish much for the diabetic patient. It focuses on both calorie counting and carb counting. The recommendation is to start out at 100g/day to 150g/day of carbohydrates. Reduce the carbohydrate intake by 10g/day for a week at a time. A target level of about 50g/day can allow the patient to adapt to the new levels sufficiently. In addition, the type of carbohydrate is equally important. Complex carbohydrates that do not spike insulin levels and metabolize more slowly are preferred, as per the glycemic index concept.

## SUPPLEMENTS FOR DIABETIC PATIENCES

Because oxidative stress contributes to diabetes and its complications, micronutrient supplementation is expected to benefit patients. It is surprising that major diabetes organizations make no supplement recommendations except in cases of known deficiency. Still, there is accumulating evidence that supplementing targeted vitamins, minerals, essential fatty acids, phytochemical antioxidants and botanicals might ameliorate these issues. These may work by one of several overlapping mechanisms: insulinotropic/sensitizing activity (e.g., chromium); blocking absorption of carbohydrate (e.g., pycnogenol); neutralizing ROS (e.g., vitamin C); inhibiting complication causing pathways (e.g., benfotiamine); or improving dyslipidemia (e.g., niacin).

When considering nutrient supplements for diabetes, few recommendations are ever suggested because ODs are often not comfortable doing so. Here are some nutrients that have proven beneficial for the diabetic patient.

- Alpha-lipoic acid (ALA): ALA is a "super antioxidant" that preferentially distributes to mitochondria. It blocks glycosylation of protein, improves glucose transport into insulin dependent tissues and reduces both small and large blood vessel complications of diabetes in animal models.

- Benfotiamine: Benfotiamine is a lipophilic analog of vitamin B1 that reduces activity in all four biochemical pathways implicated in microvascular diabetes complication.
- Chromium. Chromium potentiates the insulin receptors and consequently prevents insulin insensitivity.
- Herbal supplements. White mulberry is gaining popularity as a treatment for type 2 diabetes. This shrub has white or pinkish fruit, similar to that of a blackberry. However, it is the leaf of white mulberry that might be beneficial for diabetes. Its extract inhibits alpha-glucosidase enzymes in the gut, which prevents digestion of carbohydrates. This is similar to the mechanism of the prescription diabetes medications Precose (acarbose, Bayer Pharmaceuticals) and Glyset (miglitol, Pfizer). Evidence shows that taking 1g of white mulberry leaf powder t.i.d. for four weeks significantly reduces fasting blood glucose by about 27 percent in patients with type 2 diabetes. This is a promising holistic therapy, but more evidence is needed about long-term safety and effectiveness.
- Omega-3 essential fatty acids: Omega-3 fatty acid supplements have been shown to prevent cardiac arrhythmias and ameliorate clinical depression in type 2 diabetic patients. Several studies have demonstrated that DHA and EPA decrease amounts of plasma triglycerides, visceral fat (and concomitant production of inflammatory cytokines), free fatty acids, C-reactive protein, glucose and insulin, and they also reduce peripheral insulin resistance.
- Pycnogenol. This standardized extract of French maritime pine bark is composed of procyanidins and phenolic acids, which appear to have anti-inflammatory properties.
- Taurine. This amino acid supports glial function within the retina. Higher doses may lower blood glucose in humans.
- Vanadium. This mineral has been proven effective in the enhancement of insulin receptor site function, in turn lowering the need for constant excessive insulin production. In the absence of excess

insulin, the receptor sites work more efficiently. The end result is lowered blood sugar levels.

- Vitamin D: Vitamin D deficiency impairs insulin sensitivity and is associated with type 1 and 2 diabetes and metabolic syndrome, as well as increased risk of cancer.
- Xanthophyll carotenoids: Patients who demonstrate high levels of serum lutein/zeaxanthin and lycopene are 67 percent less likely to develop diabetic retinopathy than those with low levels.

### *Coconut Oil*

The body uses medium-chain fatty acids (MCTs) as an additional source of every. This makes coconut oil (the most common source of MCTs) a powerful means of instant energy–a function usually served in the diet by simple carbohydrates. Although coconut oil and simple carbohydrates can both deliver quick energy to the body, only coconut oil does not produce an insulin spike. It acts like a carbohydrate, but without any of the insulin-related effects associated with long-term carbohydrate consumption. Diabetics and prediabetics should immediately realize the benefit of coconut oil. In fact, coconut oil added to the diets of patients may actually help to stabilize weight gain, likely decreasing the likelihood of these patients getting type 2 diabetes.

Coconut oil also increases the activity of the thyroid, enhancing the metabolic rate. It is commonly known that a sluggish thyroid is one reason why some people are unable to lose weight, regardless of which diet they follow. Other advantages to boosting the metabolic rate include accelerated healing and an immune system that functions better overall. Because much of the saturated fat contained in coconut oil is in the form of lauric acid, coconut oil is a much better alternative to partially hydrogenated vegetable oil when a solid fat is required. While coconut oil is in a solid form at normal room temperatures, it will be in liquid form when taken into the body at 98 degrees.

## THE EYE-GUT CONNECTION

The eye-gut connection refers to the emerging understanding of the complex and bidirectional relationship between the gut microbiome and eye health. It has also been termed the gut-eye axis. This relationship suggests that the state of the gut microbiome can influence eye health, and vice versa.

Here are some key aspects of the eye-gut connection:

- *Immune Modulation*: The gut microbiota plays a critical role in shaping and regulating the immune system. Dysbiosis (an imbalance in gut bacteria) can lead to systemic inflammation, which can impact the eyes and potentially contribute to ocular diseases.
- *Production of Beneficial Metabolites*: Gut microbes produce metabolites like short-chain fatty acids (SCFAs), which have anti-inflammatory properties and can affect the eye.
- *Ocular Microbiota Influenced by Gut*: The composition of the ocular surface microbiota (OSM), the microbes residing in the eye's surface and tear film, can be influenced by the gut microbiome, indirectly impacting eye health.
- *Impact of Gut Dysbiosis*: Gut dysbiosis can be a contributing factor to various eye conditions, such as:
    - Dry Eye Disease: Gut inflammation can exacerbate ocular surface inflammation and dry eye symptoms.
    - Age-Related Macular Degeneration (AMD): Gut dysbiosis-related inflammation might accelerate AMD progression.
    - Uveitis: An autoimmune eye condition like uveitis, has been linked to gut microbiota imbalances.
    - Diabetic Retinopathy: Gut dysbiosis may worsen retinal damage in diabetic patients.

  - Glaucoma: Emerging evidence suggests a potential link between gut microbiota and optic nerve damage through neuroinflammation.

Potential therapeutic approaches based on the eye-gut connection:

- *Probiotics*: These are live microorganisms (bacteria and yeasts) that, when consumed in adequate amounts, can offer health benefits. They help restore and maintain a balanced and diverse gut microbiome, which is crucial for overall health. They can be found in fermented foods like yogurt, kefir, sauerkraut, kimchi, kombucha, and some cheeses. They are also available as dietary supplements (capsules, liquids, powders).
- *Prebiotics:* Non-digestible fibers that serve as food for beneficial gut bacteria. Specialized plant fibers that act as food for the probiotics. They are not digested by the body but serve as nourishment for the beneficial bacteria in the gut, helping them grow and thrive. These are found in fiber-rich foods like vegetables, fruits, whole grains, and legumes. Specific food examples are garlic, onions, bananas, chicory root, oats, and asparagus.
- *Postbiotics:* These are bioactive compounds and byproducts created by probiotic bacteria when they ferment prebiotics in the gut. They are live microorganisms that can help restore a healthy gut microbiome. They can have various beneficial effects on the host, such as supporting immune function, gut barrier integrity, and reducing inflammation. These are found in short-chain fatty acids (SCFAs) like butyrate, acetate, and propionate, as well as in vitamins, amino acids, and other metabolites produced during fermentation. They are naturally produced in the gut as a result of prebiotic fermentation by probiotics, and they are present in fermented foods that contain or were produced by live bacteria

- *Dietary modifications*: Focusing on a healthy, balanced diet rich in fiber and nutrients can promote a healthy gut microbiome and potentially influence eye health.
- *Fecal Microbiota Transplantation (FMT):* Transferring gut microbes from a healthy donor to a recipient to restore gut microbial balance, a potential approach being explored for some eye conditions. Obviously, a treatment option that requires a referral to a gastrointestinal specialist.

## EXERCISE MATTERS

Exercise plays an important role in diabetes management. Preventing diabetes is about lifestyle change; this includes smart dietary habits and regular physical activity. Too many individuals do not view diabetes as the serious disease that it is. On average, it shortens life by almost 10 years and significantly reduces quality of life. Individuals with high-fat diets who consume far more calories per day than they need to avoid hunger and who don't exercise at all do not seem to understand that their so-called "normal" lifestyle is slowly and literally killing them.

Muscular activity accounts for much of the body's energy consumption. Muscles also store glucose in the form of glycogen, which can be rapidly converted to glucose when energy is required for sustained, powerful contractions. Muscle cells also contain globules of fat, which are used for energy during aerobic exercise. This is why it is important to continually use those muscles—to help "burn off" the accumulation of fat!

Here are some recommendations for lifestyle change that results in more daily physical activity:

- Scheduling—Put aside a period of time every day to be used for walking and other forms of exercise. After meals, first thing in the morning, or during a mealtime (have a light lunch after your exercise session) are options; try to develop routines.

- Increasing daily activity as a lifestyle—Samples of increasing activity as part of one's daily life include taking the stairs instead of an elevator or escalator, walking instead of driving whenever possible, parking further away from your destination—not to mention lifting weights, doing calisthenics (sit-ups, push-ups), or taking a walk as a break from remaining sedentary every few hours.
- Coaching—Exercising properly is a science. Visit a fitness facility and obtain professional fitness coaching. Get tested in various measures of fitness, learn how to lift weights properly, and receive an exercise "prescription." We are motivated by numbers, so fitness tests give us the numbers for improving performance over time. Get a second test in six months to see if your fitness has improved.
- Live consistently with your values—Values are core beliefs about what you feel passionate about. What moves you? Remember what's important in your life, and try to maintain a lifestyle consistent with your values. Health, family, faith, integrity and job performance are frequent values in our culture. Are you living a life consistent with your values? If not, the inconsistencies between your values and your unhealthy habits have pretty serious consequences. Do you find the disconnection between your values and bad habits acceptable? If not, make the effort to replace those unhealthy habits with positive, more desirable routines. There are people who love you and want to see you healthy and living a long, productive, and happy life.

# THE EYE CAROTENOIDS

## *COLORING YOUR VISION*

As discussed in Part I, carotenoids are a very important contributor to eye health. Carotenoids in general are fat-soluble yellow, orange, or red pigments. To date, over 700 carotenoids have been identified in nature, but are only produced by plants, algae and bacteria. There are several sub-classifications of carotenoids, but the one most familiar are the pro-vitamin A carotenoids and the non-pro-vitamin A carotenoids, those that can and cannot be converted to vitamin A in the body. All consist of 40 carbons and contain a long linear polyene chain made of carbons connecting by alternating double bonds.

Animals appear to be incapable of biosynthesizing carotenoids, but all kinds of animals use them for a variety of purposes including coloration, and therefore they must obtain carotenoids from their diet. In humans it has been identified that about 40-50 are consumed typically in the diet but only 14 have been detected in serum. Of these, only two have been found in the retina: lutein and zeaxanthin. A third carotenoid, meso-zeaxanthin is also found in the central retina but not routinely taken in the diet.

### LUTEIN

The lutein, zeaxanthin and meso-zeaxanthin present together in the macula are known as macular pigment. Macular pigment appears as a yellow tint. The intense deposition of the yellow pigments in and around the fovea provided the basis for the clinical description of this area as the *macula lutea* or yellow spot. Macular pigment, likely via its blue light filtering property, has been shown in a number of clinical trials to enhance visual performance – the ability to perceive detailing carryout visual tasks. High levels of macular pigment contribute to improved visual acuity, glare tolerance and recovery, contrast sensitivity, chromatic aberration and photophobia in healthy individuals as well as those diagnosed with age-related eye diseases. Improvements in these parameters of visual performance can have a major impact on everyday activities. In other words, lutein and zeaxanthin act like "internal sunglasses" for the eyes.

Lutein and zeaxanthin are found naturally together in vegetables such as spinach, kale, broccoli, corn, green peas and green beans as well as other foods such as eggs. The bioavailability of lutein, unlike that of many other nutrients, is enhanced by chopping and cooking the food. This is likely due to the disruption of the strong interaction between chlorophyll and lutein molecules. It is difficult however, to obtain beneficial amounts of lutein and zeaxanthin from diet alone. Interventional studies report that 10 mg of lutein per day is effective in improving vision and reducing the risk of certain eye conditions. A survey of the standard American diet showed an approximate daily intake of 2 mg of lutein.

The ability of the macular pigment to absorb or filter blue light is measured as macular pigment optical density (MPOD). MPOD is an optical indicator of the concentration of lutein, zeaxanthin and meso-zeaxanthin in the macula is becoming an accepted biomarker not only for predicting the risk for disease but also for visual function. In numerous studies MPOD is linearly related to the levels of lutein in the serum and positively correlated with dietary intake of lutein and zeaxanthin. MPOD measurement is a relatively new technology with only a few devices commercially available to evaluate it; however, it has been well studied clinically. Dozens of studies have been published demonstrating an increase macular pigment following lutein and or zeaxanthin supplementation at a range of 2 to 30 mg per day or a high carotenoid diet. The degree of increase in MPOD levels following lutein or zeaxanthin supplementation varies, likely due to subject demographics, disease state, measurement method, diet, BMI, supplementation regimen or other factors.

There is a growing body of evidence, although not conclusive, that supports that low levels of MPOD may be a risk factor for certain age-related eye conditions. Increased levels in MPOD may provide greater protection against oxidative damage, which contributes in part to the manifestation of AMD. For example, risk factors for AMD including tobacco use, light iris color, advanced age, obesity, and female gender are associated with low levels of MPOD. Significantly less macular pigment has been found in eyes at high risk for AMD because of advanced disease in the fellow eye compared with eyes with no known risk.

SR-B1 has recently been identified as a lutein binding protein in the retina, and this same receptor plays a role in the selective uptake in the gut. In the blood, lutein is transported via high-density lipoproteins (HDL). Genes controlling SR-B1 and HDL levels predispose to AMD, which supports the involvement of cholesterol/lutein transport pathways. Apart from beneficial effects of lutein intake on various visual function tests, recent findings show that lutein can affect immune responses and inflammation. Lutein diminishes the expression of various ocular inflammation models including endotoxin induced uveitis, laser induced choroidal neovascularization, streptozotocin induced diabetes and experimental retinal ischemia and reperfusion. In vitro studies show that lutein suppresses NF kappa-B activation as well as the expression of iNOS and COX-2. Since AMD has features of a chronic low-grade systemic inflammatory response, attention to the exact role of lutein in this disease has shifted from a local effect in the eye towards a possible systemic anti-inflammatory function.

In addition to being present in the macula, lutein is also deposited in the crystalline lens, brain, and many glands, albeit at much lower concentrations. The fact that oxidation of the lens is a major contributor of cataracts suggests that antioxidant nutrients may play a role in cataract prevention. In support of this hypothesis, lutein and zeaxanthin intake from dietary sources has been linked to the reduction in risk for cataract extraction in a number of epidemiologic studies.

MPOD has the potential to become a commonly tested biomarker to measure an individual's risk for eye disease and to assess visual function knowledge of individuals MPOD level indicates whether he or she is getting enough lutein and zeaxanthin through their diet or supplementation regimen. Identification of individuals at low, medium and high risk for eye disease can be made based on their MPOD level. MPOD is typically measured on a logarithmic scale and values range from undetectable to over 1.0 optical density units (d.u.). Experts agree that the central MPOD below 0.2d.u. is considered low, between 0.2 and 0.5d.u. is midrange and levels above 0.5d.u. are high.

## ZEAXANTHIN

As often mentioned in the previous section, lutein and zeaxanthin are often mentioned together. This is due to the very similar chemical structure of the two molecules. Zeaxanthin is one of the most common carotenoid alcohols found in nature. It is the pigment that gives paprika (made from bell peppers), corn, saffron, and many other plants their characteristic color. Spirulina is also a rich source and can serve as a dietary supplement. Zeaxanthin breaks down to form picrocrocin and safranal, which are responsible for the taste and aroma of saffron.

Zeaxanthin's role is to help protect the eye from the high-energy, blue light. Zeaxanthin also protects the ganglion cells and helps the eye repair itself. In fact, studies have shown that the portion of the macula with the highest concentration of zeaxanthin is the last to degenerate. The highest density of zeaxanthin is at the very center of the macula, thus affording it the greatest protection, whereas in the peripheral retina, lutein predominates. Although there is no recommended daily intake level for zeaxanthin, a recommended amount is 8 mg daily for anyone diagnosed with macular degeneration and 2-4 mg for those taking it as a preventative measure.

Several observational studies have connected high dietary intake of foods providing zeaxanthin with lower incidence of AMD. There is currently insufficient evidence to assess the effectiveness of dietary or supplemental antioxidants in treatment or primary prevention of AMD, or the formation or progression of cataracts. Any benefit is more likely to be apparent in subpopulations of individuals exposed to high oxidative stress, such as heavy smokers or those with poor nutrition.

## MESO-ZEAXANTHIN

A third macular pigment called meso-zeaxanthin also contributes. Discovered at the Florida International University, meso-zeaxanthin is found in the retina but unlike lutein and zeaxanthin, has not been isolated from blood plasma or the liver, is not produced within the body nor derived from the traditional American diet. It can be found in shrimp shells, turtle skins and fish skin.

Meso-zeaxanthin can only be absorbed through natural conversion of enzymes from lutein. It is a powerful antioxidant, allowing greater blue light filtration as a damage preventing measure. In rare cases, there is poor conversion from lutein to meso-zeaxanthin. For these patients, supplementation of meso-zeaxanthin directly fortifies pigment density in the central macula without known adverse side effects. Due to its biochemical properties, all supplements of meso-zeaxanthin must be combined with lutein and zeaxanthin.

## OTHER CAROTENOIDS OF NOTE

### Beta-Carotene

Beta-carotene is a carotenoid, a class of compounds related to vitamin A. Some carotenoids, such as beta-carotene, can act as precursors of vitamin A. When a food or supplement containing beta-carotene is consumed, the beta-carotene is converted into vitamin A in the liver. According to recent reports, beta-carotene appears to aid in cancer prevention by scavenging, or neutralizing, free radicals. However, it should be noted that there is no beta-carotene, per se, in the eye.

Once converted into vitamin A, carotene is absorbed the same way as preformed vitamin A. The conversion of carotene into vitamin A is never 100 percent complete. Approximately one-third of the carotene in food is converted into vitamin A. Less than one-fourth of the carotene in carrots and root vegetables undergoes conversion, and about one-half of the carotene in leafy green vegetables does. Some unchanged carotene is absorbed into the circulatory system and stored in the fat tissues rather than in the liver. Unabsorbed carotene is excreted.

The degree to which carotene is utilized by the body varies with the food source and the way the food is prepared. Cooking, purĕeing, and mashing of a vegetable rupture the cell membranes and therefore make the carotene more available for absorption. Factors interfering with the absorption of vitamin A and carotene include strenuous physical activity performed within four hours of consumption of the nutrient, intake of mineral oil, excessive consumption of alcohol, excessive consumption of iron, and the use of cortisone and other medications. The intake of polyunsaturated fatty acids with carotene results in rapid destruction of the carotene unless antioxidants also are present. Even cold weather can hinder the transport and metabolism of vitamin A and carotene. Diabetics cannot convert carotene to vitamin A

Supplemental beta-carotene was shown to increase the risk of lung cancer in smokers in a poorly designed Finnish, Alpha-Tocopherol, Beta-Carotene Cancer Prevention (ATBC) study. A second study, Carotenoid and Retinol Efficacy Trial (CARET) also found a higher incidence of lung cancer in those people taking a whopping 30 mg of synthetic beta-carotene, plus 25,000 IU of preformed Vitamin A retinol.

The amount of supplemental Vitamin A and beta-carotene included in both the ATBC and CARET studies was far beyond the safe upper limits (UL) for daily consumption established by the Food and Nutrition Board at The Institute of Medicine. The UL established by The Institute of Medicine for the combination of preformed Vitamin A as retinol, and pre-formed Vitamin A as retinol activity carotenoids (primarily beta-carotene) is 10,000 IU or approximately 3,000 retinol equivalents (RAE) per day.

At about the same time, the 12-year long Physicians' Health Study (PHS), involving more than 22,000 physician volunteers, showed no statistical increase in lung cancer rates in doctors who were taking a full-spectrum multiple and 50 mg of synthetic beta carotene—even in the 11 percent of physician volunteers who were heavy smokers.

The American Journal of Epidemiology data clearly suggests that, in fact, smokers who consume small amounts of natural supplemental beta-carotene in combination with a wide variety of supplemental antioxidants actually have an overall 16 percent lower risk of developing lung and other cancer. Beta-carotene is not vitamin A. It is a rate-limiting pre-formed vitamin A hydrocarbon carotenoid. It competes with the xanthophyll carotenoids, lutein and zeaxanthin for cellular transport space, therefore excessive amounts of supplemental beta-carotene are not recommended to vision patients for that reason. The body's need for Vitamin A is so critical it will convert plant-based hydrocarbon beta-carotene to Vitamin A retinol, if and when the retinol liver stores are deficient. If there is no Vitamin A retinol deficiency, beta-carotene functions as a powerhouse antioxidant, particularly against retina-damaging singlet oxygen, and does not convert to retinol. The beta carotene/retinol conversion also becomes less efficient with the aging process; so, research-focused nutritional biochemists stopped recommending beta-carotene as a sole source of supplemental Vitamin A for older men and women years ago.

## Lycopene

Carotenoids like lycopene are important pigments found in photosynthetic pigment-protein complexes in plants, photosynthetic bacteria, fungi, and algae. They are responsible for the bright colors of fruits and vegetables, perform various functions in photosynthesis, and protect photosynthetic organisms from excessive light damage.

Lycopene is a key intermediate in the biosynthesis of many important carotenoids, such as beta-carotene and xanthophylls. Given this connection to beta-carotene and xanthophylls, many sources maintain that it is critical to eye health. However, lycopene is not modified to vitamin A in the body so it can be accessible for other benefits such as antioxidation. There is no lycopene found in the eye and any positive effect of this carotenoid to ocular health is secondary.

## Astaxanthin

Astaxanthin is a unique carotenoid that is ubiquitous in marine ecosystems. Originating in aquatic microorganisms and microalgae, astaxanthin naturally accumulates in the food chain to lend red and pink coloration to higher organisms such as krill, shrimp and salmon. Among carotenoids, astaxanthin is distinguished by a unique chemical structure, two extra hydroxyl groups. This physical nuance affords a tenfold greater antioxidant capacity than beta-carotene and lutein.

In addition to its well-established antioxidant potency, astaxanthin maintains inflammatory balance activity by modulating a central intracellular switch known as nuclear factor kappa B (NFkB). Through regulating gene expression, NFkB controls the inflammatory response in almost every cell, including those comprising the immune system, connective tissue, vascular chair, adipose tissue, eyes and skin. Accordingly, the effect of support for information with astaxanthin has been documented in clinical research.

While some references point to the positive effects of astaxanthin on ocular tissue, the emerging science on this aspect of the carotenoid is still yet to be determined. There is no astaxanthin normally residing within the structure of the eye itself. However, it does have that positive effect on striated muscle and there are six striated muscles controlling each eyeball. Thus, a powerful antioxidant that relieves muscle stress in the extraocular muscles might have an effect on the functioning of the visual system. Studies on eyestrain with computer display users have shown a positive subjective relief from digital eyestrain with low amounts of astaxanthin supplementation.

Research suggests that it may help improve blood flow by reducing oxidative stress and inflammation, which are key contributors to cardiovascular diseases. Some studies indicate that astaxanthin can lower blood pressure and improve circulation, potentially benefiting individuals at risk of heart-related conditions.

Additionally, astaxanthin has been found to support endothelial function, which plays a crucial role in maintaining healthy blood vessels. By reducing markers of inflammation and oxidative damage, it may contribute to overall heart health and better circulation. All of these effects can be amplified in ocular circulation.

## Capsanthin

One of the more recently stabilized carotenoids is capsanthin from Capsicum annum or CCA. This is different than the herb Capsaicin. Capsaicin has been proposed to have anti-obesity effects via its ability to increase energy expenditure and lipid oxidation, attenuate postprandial insulin response, increase satiety, and reduce appetite and energy intake. Capsanthin, on the other hand, is a lipophilic carotenoid, majorly found in the pericarp of ripe red pepper (*Capsicum spp.*). The greater light absorbing as well as antioxidant capacities of Capsanthin are due to the presence of eleven conjugated double bonds, a conjugated keto group, and a cyclopentane ring.

It was demonstrated that the oral administration of CapsiClear (the trade name for Capsanthin) in an animal study significantly reduced the IOP in IOP-induced rats in both eyes, even at a low dose of 20 mg/kg body weight. A beneficial effect was seen as early as ten days with treatment, and IOP returned to normal after 28 days, comparable to the vehicle-treated control groups. The IOP lowering effect of CapsiClear was similar to the effect obtained with the reference test drug, Pilocarpine.

CapsiClear was found to be safe and well-tolerated and did not result in any clinical signs of toxicity, mortality, changes in body weight, and feed consumption at all tested dose levels. There were no treatment-related changes in histopathology, hematology, and clinical chemistry parameters. Levels of critical antioxidants, such as GSH and SOD in the plasma, remained unaffected by treatment with CapsiClear. Thus, oral administration of CapsiClear in IOP-induced rats has shown to be beneficial without any adverse effects.

In this same study, it was found that administration of CapsiClear showed clinical benefits by maintaining the integrity of the corneal surface and ameliorating surface inflammation in a BAC-induced DED (dry eye) rat model. CapsiClear has a noticeable therapeutic effect on some ocular symptoms such as IOP, tear break-time, tear production, corneal inflammation, and corneal repair. CCA supplementation reduced oxidative stress by increasing glutathione peroxidase (GPX), lactoferrin (LTF), and nitric oxide (NO) production. *Capsicum annum* (CCA) could also inhibit the expressions of inflammatory cytokines, tumor necrosis factor-alpha (TNF-α), interleukins (IL-2, IL-4, IL-6), and pro-inflammatory mediator, matrix metalloproteinase 9 (MMP9), vascular cell adhesion molecule 1 (VCAM1), and prostaglandin-endoperoxide synthase 2. In summary, the research demonstrated for the first time that oral administration of CapsiClear significantly ameliorated BAC-induced DED in a rodent model. The mechanism of therapeutic action might be related to its direct inhibition of TNF-α/ IL-2/ IL-4/ IL-6 as well as MMP9, VCAM1, and PTGS2 expression.

# HERBAL THERAPY

HERBS, BY DEFINITION, ARE PLANTS THAT LACK THE WOODY CHARACTERistics of shrubs and trees. Over the years, many substances have been extracted from numerous herbs, as well as from other plants, and used successfully to heal the human body. Herbs are food for the body. They contain natural medicines, vitamins, and minerals, and have remarkable histories of curative effects when used in the proper way. Herbs have been used for centuries, and many of today's modern medicines have their foundations in herbal therapy.

The exact reasons for the positive effects that herbs exert on the human body are not always known. It is evident, however, that the nutrients stored within the plants' cellular structures are in forms that are easily metabolized by the body. The therapeutic actions of herbs come from alkaloids, organic compounds that cause certain chemical reactions within the body. Alkaloids also help the body to resist disease, strengthen tissues, and improve the nervous system. It is an often-overlooked fact that the organic chemical structures of hemoglobin and chlorophyll are very similar in molecular structure.

In this chapter, we will discuss the most popular herbs used for the eyes, as well as the most common Western herbal combinations and the traditional Chinese herbal combinations used for eye problems.

## WESTERN HERBS VS. CHINESE HERBS

Herbs are grown all over the world but some of the more popular are Chinese herbs. In China, unlike in other parts of the world, herbalists have sought out special tonic herbs that can be taken daily to improve the physical condition, enhance the energy, increase the resistance to disease, and prolong life. These herbs in particular help to distinguish Chinese herbalism from other forms of the art, such as Western herbalism. The term "Western" as used in herbalism really applies to the methods of using herbs rather than to the origins of herbs. This is why Western herb books often list substances from places such as Asia, Africa, South America, and Egypt. Individual herbs are used for their reputed health benefits, not because of the way they may act against a complex health syndrome or interact with other herbs in a combination formula.

Chinese herbalism, also known as Traditional Chinese Medicine (TCM), arranges physical signs and symptoms into patterns of organ disharmony, which can then be treated with acupuncture and herbal combinations to restore harmony and balance in the human body. The treatment of disease by TCM is generally a complicated procedure and should be performed by an experienced practitioner. The herbal formulas are often adjusted as the symptoms change during recovery. Some of these formulas are meant for short-term therapy only. There are several patented medicines made in China and the United States that can be used to treat vision problems and benefit overall health. A qualified healthcare professional, however, should oversee their use.

## FORMS OF HERBAL PREPARATIONS

Herbal preparations can be applied in many different forms. The best are the tincture and the extract, which remain potent longer than any other form. A tincture is an herb mixed in an alcohol solution. It is made by adding a powdered herb to alcohol, then adding enough water to make a 50-percent alcohol solution. Let the mixture stand for two weeks, shaking the bottle once or twice a day, then strain it before using it. An extract is made by hydraulically pressing an herb, then soaking it in alcohol or water. The excess liquid is allowed to evaporate, and the result is a concentrated liquid. Before using an extract, dilute it in a small amount of water.

***Warning: Never use an alcohol-based extract, no matter how diluted it is, directly in the eye.*** A tincture should also not be used in the eye.

Capsules are a pleasant way to take herbs, especially when the herbs taste bitter or are mucous-forming. Capsules generally consist of gelatin capsules filled with powdered herb. If prepared capsules are purchased from a first-class herb company or health food store, the herbs generally are clean and combined in the correct proportions. To comfortably wash down and properly dissolve a capsule, take it with eight ounces of pure water or herb tea.

An herbal compress will achieve an effect similar to that of an ointment, but has the advantage of the therapeutic action of heat. To make a compress, bring one or two heaping tablespoons of the herb to a boil in one cup of water. Dip a cotton pad or piece of gauze in the strained liquid, let the excess liquid drain off, and place the pad or gauze over the *closed* eyelid while still warm. Keep the compress in place until it has cooled off.

An infusion is made by pouring hot water over dry or powdered herb, and steeping the herb for several minutes to extract its active ingredients, as in brewing a tea. This method of preparation minimizes the loss of the herb's volatile elements. The usual amounts are about one-half to one ounce of herb to one pint of water. Use an enamel, stainless steel, porcelain, or glass pot with a tight-fitting lid to prevent evaporation and loss of the essential oils (the main medicinal part of some herbs). Steep the herb for about ten to twenty minutes. To drink an infusion, strain it into a cup, and drink it lukewarm or cool. For directions on how to prepare and use an infusion as eyewash, see below.

A decoction is similar to an infusion. Instead of steeping the dry herb, however, simmer it for about twenty to thirty minutes. Be careful not to boil the herb.

A poultice is a warm, mashed, moist mass of fresh or ground herb tied in a piece of muslin or other loosely woven cloth. It is applied directly to the skin to relieve inflammations, boils, and abscesses, and to promote proper cleansing and healing of the affected area. Oil the skin before applying a poultice. Because the skin around the eyes is very thin, make sure that the poultice is not too hot. A warm poultice is fine, but one that is too hot can easily cause a burn. Once a poultice has cooled, discard it. A cooled poultice should never be reheated and reused.

### Eyewashes

Having herb tea as a late-afternoon pick-me-up or just before bed to help release the tensions of the day has become as common in the United States today as tea time has been in England for centuries. But herb tea can be used as more than a drink. Used as eyewash, an herb tea infusion, or decoction can bring relief to a stressed eye through the direct application of the properties that make the herb so beneficial.

To prepare an herbal tea or other mixture for external application to the eye, use a piece of cheesecloth or filter paper, and strain the mixture repeatedly until it runs clear. In addition to being free of any debris that could scratch or irritate the eye, the mixture must also be allowed to cool to room temperature before being used. Any leftover liquid can be kept in the refrigerator for future use. However, never use a mixture that is more than two weeks old.

## THE BEST HERBS FOR THE EYES

There are many herbs that are commonly used to treat eye conditions. In the following list, they are presented according to their most popular common names, with their Latin names following. Also included is general information on each herb, what the herbs contain nutritionally, what conditions they are used to treat, and how they affect the eyes.

Most herbs can be purchased in bulk from local health-food stores or by mail order. When buying an herb, make sure that you have selected the correct variety, since quite a few herbs are known by more than one name. If you are unsure of the specific herb to buy, or of the action of an herb, consult an herbalist. It is best to store bulk herbs in airtight containers in a dark, cool place.

## Alfalfa

*Alfalfa (*Medicago sativa*)* has been used by the Chinese since the sixth century to treat kidney stones, and to relieve fluid retention and swelling. It is a perennial herb that grows throughout the world in a variety of climates. Because of its vitality and nutrient content, it is beneficial for many ailments. Alfalfa helps the body to assimilate iron, phosphorus, potassium, protein, calcium, and other nutrients. In addition, it contains high levels of chlorophyll, and therefore is a good body cleanser, infection fighter, and natural deodorizer. It also breaks down carbon dioxide.

The leaves of this legume contain eight essential amino acids. Alfalfa is a good laxative and a natural diuretic. It is useful in the treatment of urinary tract infections, and kidney, bladder and prostate disorders. Alfalfa alkalizes and detoxifies the body, especially the liver. It promotes pituitary gland function and contains an antifungus agent. Alfalfa has very rich supplies of vitamins A, D, and K. The components are properly balanced to allow for complete absorption and it is the richest land source of trace minerals.

## Bayberry

Bayberry *(Myrica cerifera)* can be useful in warding off colds at the first sign, especially when taken along with the herb capsicum *(Capsicum frutescens)*. It is also helpful when used as a gargle for tonsillitis and sore throats. It is beneficial in the rejuvenation of the adrenal glands, cleansing the bloodstream, and ridding the system of toxins. In India, the powdered root bark of bayberry is combined with ginger *(Zingiber officinale)* to successfully combat cholera. Bayberry has long been used as a tonic, stimulating the system to help raise vitality and resistance to disease, and as an aid to digestion and nutrition.

Bayberry contains a high amount of vitamin C. It kills germs, and is stimulating to the mucous membranes, especially around the eye.

## Bilberry

Bilberry *(Vaccinium myrtillus)* acts as a potent antioxidant, enhances blood circulation, has anti-inflammatory properties, and enhances the regeneration of rhodopsin in the retina. It has been shown to be completely nontoxic, with no side effects and no contraindications (except in excess as a blood thinner).

The Bilberry plant is a small shrubby perennial that grows in the woods and meadows of northern Europe. Its berries have been used for centuries to make jams and jellies, but it wasn't until after World War II that its therapeutic benefits became known. Bilberry has long been promoted as a remedy for "night blindness." This indication is not confirmed, however. Some studies show a positive effect on night vision but others have not. There have been many reports of the English RAF pilots defeating the Germans in WWII due to eating bilberry jam to see better at night. That story has not been confirmed with any authority. (Note: they also developed radar during that period).

Bilberry's fruit contains flavonoids and anthocyanin, which serve to prevent capillary fragility, thin the blood, and stimulate the release of vasodilators. This anthocyanin is a type of antioxidant that lowers blood pressure, reduces clotting and improves blood supply to the nervous system, as well as vitamins A and C, the bioflavonoids, and mineral salts. Bilberry also contains glucoquinine that has the ability to lower blood sugar.

Some of the other uses promoted for bilberry include cataracts, myopia, diabetic retinopathy, eyestrain, macular degeneration, and glaucoma. As we know, there is no one potion that heals everything, so recommend this tonic cautiously.

## Borage Oil

Borage *(Borago officinalis)* is especially soothing in cases of bronchitis and digestive upset. It promotes the activity of the kidneys and adrenal glands. It is soothing to the mucous membranes, including the conjunctiva. Borage tea can be used as an eyewash for ocular discomfort.

Borage oil contains gamma linolenic acid (GLA), a fatty acid that the body converts to prostaglandin E1 (PGE1). PGE1 has anti-inflammatory properties and may also act as a blood thinner and blood vessel dilator. Linoleic acid, a common fatty acid found in nuts and seeds and most seed oils (including borage oil), should theoretically convert to PGE1. This oil is very effective in the treatment of dry eyes.

Many things can interfere with this conversion, however, including disease, the aging process, saturated fat, hydrogenated oils (trans fats), blood sugar problems, as well as inadequate levels of vitamin C, magnesium, zinc, and B vitamins. Supplements that provide GLA circumvent these conversion problems, leading to more predictable formation of PGE1. Borage also contains calcium and potassium.

## Comfrey

Comfrey *(Symphytum officinale)* is one of the most valuable herbs known to botanical medicine. It has been used successfully for centuries as a wound healer and bone knitter. It feeds the pituitary with a natural hormone, and helps to strengthen the bones. It helps to maintain the calcium-phosphorus balance which is important for strong bones and healthy skin. It encourages the secretion of the digestive enzyme pepsin, and is a general aid to digestion. It has a beneficial effect on all the parts of the body, and is therefore used as an overall tonic. Topically, comfrey was also used to treat minor skin irritations and inflammation. It has also been used as a wash or topical application for eye irritations and for treating conjunctivitis.

Comfrey is rich in vitamins A and C. It is high in protein, calcium, phosphorus, and potassium. It contains copper, iron, magnesium, sulfur, and zinc, as well as eighteen amino acids.

Due to variations in pyrrolizidine alkaloid content, root preparations are unsafe for internal use unless they are guaranteed pyrrolizidine-free. Although comfrey root tea has been used traditionally, the danger of its pyrrolizidine alkaloids is significant. Therefore, comfrey root and young leaf preparations should not be taken internally.

## Eyebright

Eyebright (*Euphrasia officinalis*) was and continues to be used by herbalists primarily as a poultice for the topical treatment of eye inflammations, including conjunctivitis, blepharitis and styes. Traditionally, a compress made from a decoction of eyebright is used to give relief from redness and swelling due to eye infections. A tea is sometimes given internally along with the topical treatment. It has also been used for the treatment of eye fatigue and other visual disturbances of vision. In addition, herbalists have recommended eyebright for problems of the respiratory tract, including sinus infections, coughs, and sore throat.

While there are many chemicals that may be active in eyebright, none of them has been proven to have any effect on eye inflammation or irritation. Some herbal texts suggest that the astringent actions of eyebright may reduce eye irritation while others suggest that eyebright may also have antibacterial actions topically. To date, despite its name, there are no clinical studies to support or refute these proposed actions.

Eyebright aids in stimulating the liver to cleanse the blood. It is useful against inflammations because of its cooling and detoxifying properties. It has antiseptic properties that fight infections.

Eyebright is extremely rich in vitamins A and C. It contains the vitamin-B complex, vitamin D, and some vitamin E. It also has copper, iron, silicon, zinc, and a trace of iodine.

## Ginkgo Biloba

Medicinal use of Ginkgo (*Ginkgo biloba*) can be traced back almost 5,000 years in Chinese herbal medicine. The nuts of the tree were most commonly recommended and used to treat respiratory tract ailments. The use of the leaves is a modern development originating in Europe.

The medical benefits of Ginkgo biloba extract (GBE) are attributed primarily to two groups of active constituents: the ginkgo flavone glycosides and the terpene lactones. Ginkgo flavone glycosides, which typically make up approximately 24 percent of the extract, are primarily responsible for GBE's antioxidant activity and may mildly inhibit platelet aggregation. These two actions may help GBE prevent circulatory diseases, such as atherosclerosis, and support the brain and central nervous system. In addition to the cardiovascular system, GBE's antioxidant action may also extend to the brain and retina. Preliminary trials have suggested potential benefit for people with macular degeneration and diabetic retinopathy. The terpene lactones found in GBE, known as ginkgolides and bilobalide, typically make up approximately 6% of the extract. They are associated with increasing circulation to the brain and other parts of the body and may exert a protective action on nerve cells. GBE regulates the tone and elasticity of blood vessels, making circulation more efficient. However, if a person has moderate to advanced AMD, Ginkgo is contraindicated for these same reasons.

Ginkgo is also well known for its effect on memory and thinking (cognitive function). It may enhance cognitive performance in healthy older adults, in people with age-related cognitive decline, and in people with dementia or Alzheimer's disease.

## Goldenseal

Goldenseal *(Hydrastis canadensis)* has been used to boost a sluggish glandular system, and to promote youthful hormone harmony. The active ingredient of the herb goes directly into the bloodstream and helps to regulate the liver's functioning. Goldenseal has a natural antibiotic ability to stop infection and to kill poisons in the body. It is now considered an endangered species, so is used rarely by responsible herbalists. It is also very expensive.

Goldenseal is valuable against all of the mucous-forming conditions in the nasal, bronchial, throat, intestinal, stomach, and bladder areas. It has the ability to heal mucous membranes anywhere in the body, including the external eye tissue. When taken with other herbs, its tonic properties are increased for whatever ailment is being treated.

Goldenseal contains vitamins A and C. It also has the B-complex vitamins and vitamin E; the minerals calcium, copper, iron, manganese, phosphorus, potassium, sodium, and zinc; and unsaturated fatty acids.

There may be some negative interactions when taken with doxycycline or tetracycline antibiotics.

## Hawthorn

Hawthorn (*Crataegus oxycantha*) is a vasodilator that opens the blood vessels of the heart and also lowers the cholesterol level. It increases the intracellular vitamin C level, and is useful against anemia, cardiovascular and circulatory disorders, high cholesterol, and lowered immunity.

Hawthorn contains most of the B-complex vitamins and vitamin C, as well as citric acid, choline, the flavonoids, folic acid, PABA, and selenium. Hawthorne should not be taken with Digoxin.

## Marigold

Marigold *(Calendula officinalis)* is very useful as a first-aid remedy. It has been used as a tea for acute ailments, especially fevers and is effective as a tincture when applied to bruises, sprains, muscle spasms, and ulcers. It relieves earache, boosts the heart and circulation, and cleanses the lymphatic system. Traditionally, a sterile tea was topically applied in cases of conjunctivitis. Most importantly for eyecare practitioners is that the most common source of lutein in the US is marigold flowers.

Marigold is high in phosphorus, and contains vitamins A and C. Flavonoids, found in high amounts in calendula, are thought to account for much of its anti-inflammatory activity. Other potentially important constituents include the triterpene saponins and carotenoids (specifically lutein and zeaxanthin). Many of the companies that source lutein and zeaxanthin use marigold flowers as the source. The saponins are sugars that can be easily cleaved off in the gut by bacteria, allowing them to be inserted into cell membranes, where they can modify the composition, influence membrane fluidity, and potentially affect signaling by many ligands and cofactors. Saponin glycosides reduce surface tension of water with foaming and will break down lipids.

## Passionflower

Passionflower *(Passiflora incarnata)* is used to treat insomnia and hysteria, as well as hyperactivity and convulsions in children. It is an herb that is quieting and soothing to the nervous system, and should be recommended to patients who wish to wean themselves from synthetic sleeping pills or tranquilizers. Passionflower helps to reduce high blood pressure and tachycardia, and is an effective antispasmodic. It is good for inflamed eyes. Passionflower contains bioflavonoids, so exhibits anti-cancer and anti-diarrheal activities.

## Red Clover

Red clover *(Trifolium pratense)* is useful as a tonic for the nerves and as a sedative for nervous exhaustion. Native Americans used the plant for sore eyes and as a salve for burns. It is useful when mixed with honey and water as a cough syrup. It is also good as an aid for strengthening the immune systems of delicate children. Red clover is effective against coughs, a weak chest, wheezing, bronchitis, lack of vitality, and nervous energy. It has also been included in some well-known cancer mixtures.

Red clover is a good source of vitamin A. It is high in iron, and contains the B-complex vitamins, vitamin C, the bioflavonoids, and unsaturated fatty acids. It is valued for its high mineral content. For example, it is rich in calcium, copper, and magnesium, and contains some cobalt, manganese, nickel, selenium, sodium, and tin.

## Rose Hips

Rose hips *(Rosa canina)* are the fruit of a rose that develop after the petals have fallen. They are very nourishing to the skin. Rose hips contain a natural fruit sugar. They help to prevent infections, and also help when an infection has already developed.

Rose hips are very high in the vitamin-B complex, and are very rich in vitamins A, C, and E. (It is the herb with the highest Vitamin C content). They also contain vitamin D and the bioflavonoids. Rose hips are high in calcium and iron. They also have some potassium, silica, sodium, and sulfur.

## Rosemary

Rosemary *(Rosmarinus officinalis)* is a stimulant, especially of the circulatory system and pelvic region. It is considered a proven heart tonic, and is a treatment for high blood pressure. Rosemary is used externally on bites and stings. In cases of colds or flu, it can be taken in the early stages as a warm infusion, and may be used as a cooling tea when the symptoms include restlessness, nervousness, and insomnia. It has been considered one of the most powerful remedies to strengthen the nervous system. Rosemary is a good tonic for the reproductive organs. It has also been effective against diarrhea, especially in children.

Rosemary contains vitamins A and C. It is high in calcium, and also contains iron, magnesium, phosphorus, potassium, sodium, and zinc.

## Rue

Rue *(Ruta graveolens)* has the ability to expel poisons from the system, and therefore has been used for snake, scorpion, spider, and jellyfish bites. It helps to remove deposits that tend to form in the tendons and joints with age, especially in the wrist joints. It has also been found to be effective at treating high blood pressure, and helps to harden the bones and teeth.

Rue contains a large amount of rutin. Rutin is a bioflavonoid that is known for its ability to strengthen the capillaries, arteries and veins. It is also commonly used in its homeopathic form.

## Sarsaparilla

Sarsaparilla *(Smilax officinalis)* is a valuable herb used in glandular-balancing formulas. Its stimulating properties are noted for increasing the metabolic rate. Sarsaparilla also contains precursors of both the male and female hormones. It has been used to relieve sore eyes, but the specifics of the mechanism of action has yet to be determined.

Sarsaparilla contains vitamins A, B-complex, C, and D. It also has copper, iodine, iron, manganese, silicon, sodium, sulfur, and zinc.

## Siberian Ginseng

Siberian ginseng *(Eleutherococcus)* is very effective at increasing the circulation, especially around the heart; normalizing the blood pressure; and combating stress and fatigue. It increases brain and physical efficiency and improves the concentration span. It also strengthens the adrenal and reproductive glands. Siberian ginseng contains the B-complex vitamins, vitamin E, and eleutherosides, a type of complex sugar molecule with beneficial effects.

It also stimulates T-cell production (supports the immune system) and improves blood lipid levels. It is a powerful antioxidant.

## Taheebo

Taheebo *(Tabebuia)* also goes by the names: pau d'arco, lapacho, and ipe roxo. It is found in South America, and is a very powerful antibiotic with virus-killing properties. Taheebo is said to contain compounds that seem to attack the causes of diseases. One of its main actions purportedly is to put the body into a defensive posture, to give it the energy needed for defense against and resistance to disease.

Taheebo contains a high amount of iron, which aids in the proper assimilation of nutrients and the elimination of wastes. Considering that, caution should be the rule when recommending this herb to men and non-menstruating women.

## Wild Cherry

Wild Cherry (*Prunus serotina*) is considered to be a very useful expectorant. It is a valuable remedy for all mucous-forming conditions, and is beneficial against bronchial disorders caused by hardened accumulations of mucous. Wild cherry contains a volatile oil that acts as a local stimulant in the alimentary canal and aids digestion. It is a useful tonic for persons convalescing from various chronic diseases.

Wild Cherry Bark is believed to possess antioxidant properties that may be helpful in the fight against the oxidative damage to cells and tissues. Its amygdalin content is believed to be the active constituent responsible for this effect.

## HERBS TO AVOID

As much as we can reap positive effects from herbal remedies, we also need to take some precautions in their use. If patients are taking medications for certain diseases, some herbs may interfere with their activity or efficacy. For example, the following herbs have the same anti-inflammatory effect as steroids—and can cause the same ocular problems, such as cataracts, glaucoma, herpes simplex keratitis, light sensitivity, and retinal blood vessel problems:

| | |
|---|---|
| Beetroot | Damiana |
| Fenugreek | Ginseng |
| Licorice | Saw palmetto |
| Blue cohosh | False unicorn root |
| Figwort | Goldenrod |
| Red sage | Wild yam |

There are also some herbs that have the same effects as aspirin (salicylates), as well as the same ocular effects of blurred vision, disturbed accommodation, optic atrophy, retinal edema and visual field constriction. These herbs are:

| | |
|---|---|
| Birch | Sweet violet |
| Chickweed | Black willow |
| Pansy | Meadowsweet |
| Black cohosh | Wintergreen |
| Cramp bark | Blue flag |

Diuretics are substances that affect the fluid and electrolyte balances in the body. They can cause blurred vision, disturbed accommodation, dry eyes, light sensitivity, xanthopsia and myopia. Herbs that act as diuretics are:

| | | |
|---|---|---|
| Bearberry | Shepherd's purse | Couch grass |
| Buchu | Parsley | Juniper |
| Birch | Stone root | Dandelion |
| Bugleweed | Corn silk | Licorice |
| Blue flag | Sweet violet | Fumitory |
| Carline thistle | Saw palmetto | Night blooming cereus |
| Boldo | Wild carrot | Gravel root |
| Cleavers | Sea holly | Pansy |
| Broom tops | Yarrow | Hydrangea |

Some herbs contain volatile or aromatic oils that can cause ocular effects such as excessive tearing, irritation, contamination of contact lenses, and disorders of the central nervous system. These herbs are:

| | | |
|---|---|---|
| Cinnamon | Fennel | Peppermint |
| Rosemary | Tansy | Wild carrot |
| Clove | Garlic | Prickly ash |
| Selfheal | Thuja | Willow |
| Cudweed | Ginger | Queen's delight |
| Skunk cabbage | Thyme | Wintergreen |
| Echinacea | Pennyroyal | Red sage |
| Southernwood | Valerian | |

Some herbs have a drying effect on the eye tissue. This can, in some cases, be detrimental, especially if you have a dry eye condition or are wearing contact lenses. Some of these drying herbs are:

| Bistort | Cudweed |
|---|---|
| Eyebright | Golden seed |
| Mouse ear | Pokeroot |
| Coltsfoot | Daisy |
| Golden root | Ground ivy |
| Myrrh | Scots pine |

Other herbs and their possible side effects are:

Arnica—eye irritation

Bittersweet—blurred vision, dilated pupils, loss of accommodation, glaucoma, light sensitivity

Bladderwrack—metabolic changes due to altered thyroid activity

California poppy—constricted pupils

Canthaxanthin—abnormalities in visual field, retina function and dark adaptation

Chamomile—severe conjunctivitis

Datura—dilated pupils

Echinacea—eye irritation, conjunctivitis

Ephedra—dilated pupils, dry eyes, increased eye pressure

Ginkgo Biloba—retinal hemorrhage

Kava—blurred vision, redness, dilated pupils

Licorice—transient visual loss

Shepherd's purse—blurred vision, red eyes, constricted pupils

Squill, figwort, hawthorn, lily of the valley, night blooming cereus—lazy eye, blurred vision, central blind spot, double vision, disturbed color vision, disturbed accommodation, light sensitivity.

Herbs are naturally occurring substances in nature that have medicinal-type actions on our bodies. We can use herbs to treat disease, avoiding many of the negative side effects of medications. But like medications, herbs can also be harmful if taken inappropriately. Therefore, you should take care when choosing an herbal therapy. I strongly recommend consulting a qualified herbalist to discuss your options before taking or recommending any herb for any reason.

## HERBAL COMBINATIONS FOR EYE PROBLEMS

Herbal combinations have more than one function in the fight against eye problems; since they consist of several substances that each has their own benefits and that work together in natural harmony. When taken over a period of time, an herbal combination will condition the body to react in a way that is comparable to the effects produced by certain medications, but in a less drastic manner and often without the unwanted side effects. This is because the herbs trigger neuro-chemical reflexes in the body that over time become automatic and continue even after the person stops taking the herbs. One advantage of using an herbal combination instead of a medication is that the herbs help the body to bring about its own recovery and make it unlikely to be susceptible to the same complaint during or after convalescence. Unlike medications, which treat symptoms, herbal combinations go right to the root of the disorder and treat its cause.

Two herbal combinations that work especially well for the eyes:

*Herbal Combination Number One*, which consists of the following herbs:

Bayberry—high in vitamin C; kills germs; stimulates the mucous membranes.

Eyebright—may boost the body's immunity to eye problems.

Goldenseal—acts as a natural antibiotic against eye infections.

Bayberry, eyebright, and goldenseal are three of the more common herbs used for external eye conditions. Although each one used separately is effective, the combination benefits several types of eye conditions, which make this combination a good choice if you are not sure of exactly what is wrong with the patient's eyes. Specifically, this combination might be good for cataracts, iritis, conjunctivitis and night blindness.

> *Herbal Combination Number Two* consists of the three herbs from Herbal Combination Number One plus the following herbs:
>
> Raspberry—effective against styes; astringent action helps to stop discharge.
>
> Capsicum—acts as a stimulant and a relaxant; high in vitamin A and a number of minerals.

Use caution with Herbal Combination Number Two. Capsicum is a very powerful herb and can cause severe damage to delicate tissues if not used properly. If the eye is very inflamed and has a discharge, use a very small amount of capsicum in the mixture. This combination will help to increase the circulation in the eye area to rid the tissue of toxins. Consult an herbalist if you have any concerns or questions about the proper combination of herbs to use.

When using an herbal combination, follow the same precautions outlined for single herbs at the beginning of this section. A number of pre-mixed herbal combinations are available from health food stores and by mail order, but you can also mix a combination yourself if you are careful to keep your ingredients, tools, and work area clean. The usual recipe calls for approximately equal amounts of the different herbs. To prepare a tea, infusion, or other desired mixture, follow the procedures described for single herbs in "Forms of Herbal Preparations" (beginning of this section).

## TRADITIONAL CHINESE HERBAL COMBINATIONS FOR EYE PROBLEMS

Chinese medicine is a science and art form that is well over 5,000 years old. The procedures and symptomology of Chinese medicine differ significantly from those of Western medicine. For example, a Chinese medical practitioner generally asks different types of questions and performs different diagnostic tests than does a Western medical practitioner. The emotional aspects of illness are often of more concern to Chinese practitioners than to Western practitioners, and Chinese and Western practitioners often find different patterns in the health of the patient to be of interest. Oftentimes, there is no correlation between our Western medical terminology and diagnoses, and those of traditional Chinese medicine.

Some of the traditional Chinese herbal combinations contain herbs chosen because of the way they interact with one another. It is rare for Chinese practitioners to use one herb alone. Some combinations include as many as twenty-five different herbs. A number of combinations also include non-herbal ingredients, such as minerals, plants, and animal organs. Therefore, many of the combinations in the following list are not used strictly for eye conditions. Since Chinese medicine strives to treat the whole person—the body, mind, and spirit—the treatment oftentimes is also directed toward a whole other set of symptoms, which may or may not be apparent.

The Chinese use their observations of nature to describe the workings of the inner body. For example, if a practitioner talks about "heat from the liver," he or she may be describing a series of conditions caused by an emotional constraint or blockage of energy in the liver. This "heat from the liver" may manifest as an inflammation (a Western medical term) in the head area—for example, a sore throat, earache, red eyes, or irritability. A person's condition is a very individualized expression of a disorder, and different people may display completely different combinations of symptoms. The different combinations of symptoms that are possible are what have given rise to the various herbal combinations used in traditional Chinese medicine.

Some of the more common traditional Chinese herbal combinations that may have beneficial effects on eye conditions are the following:

| Chinese Herb | Effects |
|---|---|
| *An mian pian* | This combination cools liver "heat." The symptoms it helps to relieve include anxiety, red eyes, and eye irritation. |
| *Er ming zuo ci wan* | This combination is used to treat a liver deficiency that is causing symptoms such as headaches, high blood pressure, eye pressure, insomnia, thirst, and eye irritation. |
| *Long dan xie gan wan* | This is the classic combination for purging liver and gallbladder "heat." Use it for headaches; red, burning eyes; ringing in the ears; sore throat; fever blisters on the mouth; scanty urination; and constipation. |
| *Ming mu di huang wan* | This combination replenishes the energy in the liver and kidneys. The symptoms it can be used for include dry eyes; red, itchy eyes; poor eyesight; light sensitivity; excessive tearing; and eye diseases such as glaucoma and cataracts. |
| *Ming mu shang qing pian* | This combination dispels "heat," clears the vision, and sedates the liver. Use it for liver "heat" that is affecting the eyes, causing redness, itching, tearing, and swelling. |
| *Nei zhang ming yan wan* | This combination benefits the clarity of vision, nourishes the liver and kidneys, reduces "heat," and helps the circulation. Use it when vision is impaired due to a liver deficiency, to aid recovery from eye surgery, and for cataracts, glaucoma, disturbed clarity of vision and itchy, painful eyes. |
| *Niu huang shang qing wan* | Use this combination for systemic "heat" rising from the liver, causing headaches, eye pain or red eyes, sore throat, toothache, or a fever with thirst. |
| *Qi ju di huang wan* | This combination nourishes the kidneys, boosting their energy. The symptoms it helps include blurred vision; dry, painful eyes; pressure behind the eyes; and disturbed night vision. It can also be used for dizziness, headaches, pain behind the eyes and restlessness. |

(*continued*)

| Chinese Herb | Effects |
|---|---|
| *Shi hu ye guang wan* | This combination improves vision, especially eyesight that is beginning to become blurry or is affected by dizziness. It is valuable in the early stages of cataract formation. It is also suitable for use with tearing eyes, red or itchy eyes, dry eyes, or hypertensive changes within the eyes. |
| *Xiao yao wan* | This is a basic combination for stagnation of the liver due to a blood deficiency. The symptoms it relieves are diverse and include digestive dysfunction, menstrual and premenstrual disorders, vertigo, headaches, fatigue, blurred vision, and red, painful eyes. It is also useful for treating food allergies, chronic hay fever, and hypoglycemia. |
| *Zhong guo shou wu zhi* | This combination is an excellent tonic for the blood. It nourishes the liver and kidneys, and benefits the eyes and tendons. |

Since herbal preparations are not "pure" substances, you need to use caution when taking them. The problem is that different parts of the herbs—the roots, leaves, pods, bark, seeds, flowers—are often used, giving different batches varying degrees of potency, or strength. In some cases, the potency of the active ingredient in an herb matches or exceeds that of the medication manufactured using that ingredient. Furthermore, some companies package and market their products in a way that fosters misuse of natural products by consumers who believe that natural equals weak and safe. And, of course, some products do have undesirable side effects, which can lead to dire consequences. I highly recommend consultation with an experienced herbalist before taking any herb or herbal combination.

In short, it's best to leave prescribing Chinese herbs to practitioners who have studied them specifically and know how they work best.

# HOMEOPATHY

Homeopathy (ho-me-OP-a-thee) is a system of medicine whose principles are even older than Hippocrates. It seeks to cure in accordance with the natural laws of healing, and uses medicines made from natural animal, vegetable, and mineral substances. These remedies are prepared in such a way that they are nontoxic and do not cause side effects.

Homeopathic medicines are prescribed according to an age-old principle that recognizes the body's ability to heal itself. This is not a new approach to healing. This approach was "discovered" in the early 1800s by a German physician named Samuel Hahnemann. It was extremely popular in the United States in the nineteenth century, then declined because of the new "wonder drugs" and other political and economic changes in the practice of medicine. The holistic movement that surfaced in the early 1970s has been advocating a return to the natural laws of healing and has sparked a revival of interest in this scientific system of medicine.

Because you may not be familiar with the process used to produce homeopathic remedies and the system of diagnosis and treatment, we will describe the laws of homeopathy in this chapter. We also will discuss the specific remedies that can be used to help the eyes and the visual system.

## THE LAWS OF HOMEOPATHY

Like any science, the system of homeopathy is governed by certain "laws" that dictate how the process works. These laws must be followed in order for the process to be considered homeopathic. These laws are called the "Law of Similars", the "Law of Proving", and the "Law of Potentization".

## The Law of Similars

The term "homeopathy" comes from the Greek *homoios* ("similar") and *pathos* ("suffering" or "sickness"). The fundamental law upon which homeopathy is based is called the Law of Similars, which states that "like is cured by like." According to the Law of Similars, a remedy can cure a disease if it produces, in a healthy person, symptoms that are similar to those of the illness.

The basic concept of the Law of Similars is attributed to Hindu sages from the tenth century B.C., who described the law as, "Through the like, disease is produced, and through the application of the like, it is cured." The following is an example of how the law works: A person develops a fever, with a flushed face, dilated pupils, rapid heartbeat, and feeling of restlessness. Their homeopathic physician studies all these symptoms, then searches for a remedy that, under scientifically controlled conditions, has produced all these symptoms in a healthy person. Within a short time after taking the remedy, the man's fever drops to normal, and he begins to feel well again. In other words, using the Law of Similars, a doctor selects the one medicine needed by the patient by matching the symptoms of the patient's disorder to the symptoms the remedy is known to induce.

## The Law of Proving

The second law of homeopathy, the Law of Proving, refers to the method used to test a substance to determine its medicinal effect. To prove a remedy, half of a group of healthy people is given a dose of the test substance, and the remaining half is given a placebo (an inactive substance). Conforming to the standard double-blind method used in pharmacological experiments, neither the subjects nor the researchers know which substance a particular person is taking. Every day, all the subjects carefully record the symptoms they experience. When the proving is complete, it is determined who took what, and all the symptoms experienced by the persons taking the substance are listed as a characteristic remedy picture in the reference book. To treat a patient, a physician looks up the remedy picture in the reference book, and, when the symptoms fit, applies the Law of Similars.

## The Law of Potentization

The third law of homeopathy, the Law of Potentization, refers to the method of preparation of a homeopathic remedy. All homeopathic remedies are prepared using a controlled process consisting of dilution followed by succussion (shaking), which may be repeated until the resulting medicine contains few or no molecules of the original substance. These dilutions are called potencies. Lesser dilutions are known as low potencies, and greater dilutions are known as high potencies. As strange as it may seem, the more a remedy is diluted, the greater is its potency. The potencies are designated by a number followed by an "x" or "c." The "x" represents 10, and signifies that the original tincture has been diluted to 1 part in 10. The "c" represents 100, and signifies that the original tincture has been diluted to 1 part in 100. The original tincture is an alcohol-based extract of the substance as it comes directly from the plant, animal, or mineral. The number preceding the "x" or "c" indicates the number of times the remedy has been diluted. Thus, a 3x-potency remedy has been diluted three times, and a 6x-potency remedy has been diluted six times. For purposes of consistency, the recommended homeopathic remedies in this book are all 6x and should be used three to four times daily.

When the process of potentization was devised roughly 200 years ago, the idea that medicine containing an infinitesimal amount of matter could be curative was inconceivable. In this nuclear age, however, the power of minute quantities is all too well established. The dose of vitamin B12 that is used to treat certain anemias contains one-millionth of a gram of cobalt. Trace elements, essential for physical development and functioning, are present in the body in barely measurable amounts. The human body manufactures only fifty- to one-hundred-millionth of a gram of thyroid hormone each day, yet a small deviation in the amount can seriously affect the health of an individual.

The power of the infinitesimal dose is not clearly understood, but neither are the actions of many modern medications. The process of potentization makes it possible to use as medicines substances such as certain metals, charcoal, and sand, which are inert in their natural states.

Potentized remedies do not contain sufficient matter to act directly on the tissues, which means that homeopathic medicines are nontoxic and cannot cause side effects.

## SINGLE REMEDIES

Contrary to the current medical practice of prescribing two or more medicines for use at the same time, most homeopaths usually recommend only one remedy at a time. It is unknown what the effect of using two remedies would be, but the effects of using a single remedy are well known. Single remedies have been proved, or tested, on healthy subjects.

Many homeopathic remedies are sold today in health food stores under the description of the symptoms, for example, "Colds," "Flu," or "Teething." These are combination remedies and may be as effective as single remedies, but probably are not.

| COMMON HOMEOPATHIC REMEDIES | |
|---|---|
| **Remedy** | **Indications** |
| Aconite | For any kind of pain or injury. |
| Agaricus | For dimmed vision. |
| Allium cepa | For headaches, mostly in the forehead area. |
| Anacardium | For swollen eyes. |
| Antimonium crudum | For eyelid inflammation. |
| Apis mellifica | For bee stings; puffy swelling around the eyes. |
| Argentum nitricum | For sticky eyelids. |
| Arnica montana | For eye injuries; black eyes; any kind of bruising. |
| Arsenicum album | For the late stages of head colds; red eyes; foggy vision. |
| Aurum | For any kind of pain; double vision. |
| Belladonna | For dilated pupils; red eyes; light sensitivity. |
| Bryonia | For headaches; dry, hard coughs. |
| Calcarea fluorica | For the appearance of flickering lights. |

| Remedy | Indications |
|---|---|
| Calcarea sulfurica | For discharge from any kind of infection. |
| Calendula officinalis | For general dryness associated with irritants. |
| Carboneum sulfuratum | For any kind of swelling. |
| Causticum | For purifying any kind of tissue. |
| Chamomilla | For calming any kind of tissue. |
| Cinchona officinalis | For dilated pupils. |
| Cineraria maritima | For red, irritated eyes. |
| Cocculuc | For floaters. |
| Conium | For the heavy-eye feeling. |
| Cyclamen | For tense eye muscles. |
| Euphrasia officinalis | For any kind of burning and irritation. |
| Ferrum phosphoricum | For the early stage of any kind of inflammation; red eyes. |
| Gelsemium sempervirens | For tired eyes; aching all over the body. |
| Glonoinum | For red eyes. |
| Graphites | For light sensitivity. |
| Hyoscyamus | For double vision. |
| Hypericum perforatum | For eye injuries; any kind of shooting pain. |
| Ignatia amara | For severe headaches; emotional stress. |
| Kali muriaticum | For the "gritty" feeling in eyes. |
| Kali sulfuricum | For red eyes. |
| Lac caninum | For blurred vision. |
| Lachesis | For dull vision. |
| Ledum palustre | For eye pain if Arnica montana fails to relieve it. |
| Lycopodium | For eye pain; tearing. |
| Magnesia carbonica | For red, inflamed, burning eyes. |
| Magnesia phosphorica | For a general feeling of tiredness; double vision. |
| Mercurius corrosivus | For eye discharge. |
| Mercurius vivus | For swollen glands; red eyes with no discharge. |
| Natrum muriaticum | For eye pain. |

(*continued*)

| **COMMON HOMEOPATHIC REMEDIES (*con't*)** | |
|---|---|
| **Remedy** | **Indications** |
| Natrum sulfuricum | For light sensitivity. |
| Nitricum acidum | For tearing. |
| Nux vomica | For light sensitivity; headaches. |
| Petroleum | For eyelid inflammation. |
| Physostigma | For tense eye muscles. |
| Pulsatilla | For sticky eyelids; yellowish discharge. |
| Rheum | For any kind of muscle twitching. |
| Rhus toxicodendron | For light sensitivity; tearing. |
| Ruta graveolens | For eyestrain followed by headache; red eyes. |
| Sanguinaria | For eye pain. |
| Senecio | For any kind of muscle weakness. |
| Sepia | For excessive tearing. |
| Silicea | For eye pain accompanied by light sensitivity. |
| Spigelia | For eye pain. |
| Staphysagria | For any kind of infection. |
| Stramonium | For dilated pupils. |
| Sulphur | For red eyelids. |
| Symphytum | For injuries to the eyeball; pain from a blow to the eye. |
| Veratrum album | For dry eyes; cold sweats. |
| Zincum metallicum | For general dryness; foggy vision. |

As you can see, there can be many different remedies for the same symptoms. That is why a series of questions must be answered to determine which specific remedy is most appropriate for your condition. This type of approach takes extensive training and should only be applied by a homeopathic physician or specialist.

## HOMEOPATHY VS. HERBALISM

Many people are confused about the differences between homeopathy and herbalism because both systems use herbs as medicines. The methods of preparing the remedies are very different, however. An herbalist may use an age-old formula for making an herb tea or a poultice, but can also improvise like a cook, personalizing the recipe. In addition, using intuition and experience, herbalists often combine a number of herbs to increase the effect desired. Homeopathy is somewhat more scientific, its remedies prepared, tested, and prescribed according to specific laws and procedures.

Some herbs, by themselves, are toxic, particularly when they are ingested in large amounts. Herbalists cannot use these herbs. Although many homeopathic remedies are made from poisonous herbs or plants, the potentized remedies contain only minute amounts of the original substances and are nontoxic. It cannot be overemphasized that caution should be taken with any self-remedy. Although a homeopathic remedy may be harmless because of its low potency, it can also be ineffective at treating a disorder. This is why it is important to work in conjunction with a trained homeopathic physician.

### Homeopathy and the Eyes

Although we have been emphasizing that the eyes are an integral part of the body and, like the body, respond to nutritional influences and environmental factors, there are not very many homeopathic remedies specifically for the disorders that afflict them. The remedy may not be directed at the specific eye disorder or even at the chief complaint, but at the person as a whole. The correct remedy may act instantaneously, like an electric spark, upon the defense mechanism or vital force; and the effects of one dose may last for a month.

Homeopathic remedies come in pellets, tablets, creams and liquids. The liquid form is an alcohol-based extract of a specific remedy and therefore should not be used directly on the eye. The liquid generally is placed under the tongue with an eyedropper, which usually comes with the bottle. The liquid can also be used to make a cream, ointment, or salve, which is done by mixing the liquid with a cream or gel base. Creams, ointments, and salves are almost never used on the eye tissue itself. Tablets and pellets, which are made with a base of lactose (sweet milk sugar), are dissolved in the mouth, usually under the tongue, without chewing. They are excellent for use with children. However, they should not be touched, as this may decrease their effectiveness. For infants, dissolve a pellet or tablet in water and administer it to the child using an eyedropper. Since the oral liquid remedies contain alcohol, they should be given to children only in small doses.

The best time to take a homeopathic treatment is thirty minutes before or after eating. Strong flavors such as mint or camphor, odors from perfumes and paints, and caffeine are believed to decrease the effectiveness of homeopathic remedies. Homeopathy requires personal observation to determine the length of treatment. If no change occurs in a chronic ailment after a week, switch to another remedy. If improvement is noted, continue with the remedy until all the symptoms disappear. It is very important to continually be aware of the symptoms because the remedy should be changed as the symptoms change. For example, a sore throat may turn into a headache, which may turn into sneezing or coughing, which may lead to a runny nose. Each of these symptoms has a separate remedy that is specific for that symptom. For a list of common homeopathic remedies and the symptoms for which they can be used, see the table on page XX.

Homeopathic treatment is different from traditional Western medicine in many ways. Homeopathic remedies treat the series of symptoms as unique, without necessarily assigning a "syndrome" name to the condition. Patients might be tempted to try to treat their own symptoms based on the conditions listed in this book and the remedies given for each. However, a homeopathic practitioner may see a whole other set of symptoms, based on further questioning, that might indicate they should take a different remedy. He or she will also take your physical characteristics, personality, and emotional state into consideration. It is best to consult a trained homeopathic practitioner before attempting any treatment on your own patients.

# DRUG-NUTRIENT INTERACTIONS

MANY PATIENTS SEEM TO FORGET THAT THEY ARE TAKING VITAMINS and minerals, especially when filling out case history forms. When asked about "pills or medications", they'll likely not consider listing any vitamin or mineral supplement. Even if they do recall that they are taking them, they may consider the fact inconsequential or they may actively hide that fact to their doctor. The rationale may be that they are "only" vitamins and don't figure into their health visit.

However, treating nutritional supplements casually or keeping them a secret from a physician could be a mistake. Some medications are known to interact with minerals or vitamins in a negative manner, but you probably won't think to give the patient advice on avoiding these dangers unless you know that they are taking them. The popularity of vitamin and mineral supplements has increased dramatically over the past decade or so as baby boomers look to remain healthy. With more and more people taking vitamin pills, the potential for interactions with popular drugs also increases.

Unfortunately, researchers have not devoted significant time and energy to the study of how nutrients interact with drugs, partly because the practical benefits are not immediately apparent. The FDA has not required drug companies to spend the time or resources required to uncover such interactions. The chart listed below summarizes information on how drugs affect nutrient status and nutritional supplements may interfere with optimal drug benefits. This field is still evolving and we expect more information become available over the next several years. Please remember to ask your patients about their vitamin and mineral intake.

| Drug | Nutrient | Interaction |
|---|---|---|
| Acne Medicine (Accutane) | Vitamin A | Because Accutane is related to vitamin A, taking these two compounds together could increase toxicity. Avoid this combination |
| Alcohol | Beta-Carotene<br><br>Folic Acid/ Thiamine<br><br><br><br>Vitamin B6; Vitamin B12; Vitamin C; Iron; Zinc | Beta-carotene can increase the liver damage caused by chronic alcohol intake.<br>One consequence of long-term alcohol abuse is brain damage. Lack of the B vitamin thiamine plays an important role in the development of this problem.<br>Absorption or utilization of vitamins B6, B12, and C is affected by regular alcohol intake. In addition, traders may absorb too much iron and too little sleep |
| Antacids | Calcium Phosphate<br><br><br><br><br>Thiamine | The aluminum and magnesium and antacids can form a complex with phosphate and deplete the body of calcium. Anyone at risk of osteoporosis should be cautious about this interaction.<br>Aluminum-based antacids may inactivate thiamine. Don't take them at mealtime. |
| Antibiotics | Vitamin K | Broad-spectrum antibiotics can mess up the good intestinal bacteria that make vitamin K. In some cases this could lead to unusual bleeding. |
| Fluoro-quinolones | Calcium; Iron; Zinc | These antibiotics may not work as well as expected if they are taken at the same time and certain minerals. This includes antacids as well as nutritional supplements. |

| Drug | Nutrient | Interaction |
|---|---|---|
| Tetracyclines | Calcium; Iron; Magnesium; Riboflavin; Vitamin C; Zinc | Calcium and other minerals can combine with tetracyclines so that the antibiotics are not absorbed into the body. Make sure patients don't take any mineral supplements or mineral containing antacids within two hours of a tetracycline pill. Long-term use of tetracycline may deplete these nutrients and require supplementation. |
| Arthritis medicines (analgesics) | Vitamin C | Aspirin may block vitamin C from getting into cells. |
| | Folic Acid | Folic acid levels are lower when people rely on large doses of aspirin. Regular users may need a folic acid supplement. |
| | Iron | Small amounts of blood are regularly lost from the stomach when aspirin is taken. This can add up over time and deplete the body of iron while this can actually be beneficial for people at risk of heart disease, be cautious of iron anemia. A blood test is needed for diagnosis. |
| Iindomethacin | Iron | Indomethacin irritates the stomach lining even more than aspirin. Over time, continued low-level blood loss could lead to iron deficiency. |
| Methotrexate | Folic Acid; Vitamin B12; Beta-Carotene | Methotrexate affects the intestinal wall so that these nutrients are not absorbed efficiently. Nutritional imbalances may result. |
| Penicillin | Iron; Magnesium; Copper; Zinc; Vitam n B6 | Penicillin may not be well absorbed if it is taken at the same time as iron ore magnesium. This medicine may also deplete the body of copper or zinc, causing a loss of the sense of taste. |

(*continued*)

| Drug | Nutrient | Interaction |
|---|---|---|
| Birth Control Pills | Vitamin B6; Folic Acid; Vitamin E<br><br>Vitamin C | Women using combination oral contraceptives may need more of these vitamins both folic acid and B6 levels may be low and too little vitamin B6 could be responsible for depression.<br>Vitamin C may increase blood levels of estrogen. |
| Blood Pressure Medicines | Potassium | Popular blood pressure medications tend to maximize potassium levels. This is fine unless the person is getting extra potassium through a potassium supplement or a potassium-based salt substitute too much of this important mineral is just as bad as not enough. |
| Diuretics | Calcium; Magnesium; Potassium | Diuretics may cause the loss of important minerals from the body. Periodic blood tests are essential to see whether supplements are needed. |
| Blood Thinners | Vitamin C<br><br>Vitamin E<br><br>Vitamin K | Very large amounts of vitamin C (5 g or more) could interfere with the effectiveness of these medications.<br>Vitamin E itself acts as an anticoagulant in the combination may thin the blood too much and lead to bruises or excessive bleeding.<br>Vitamin K counteracts these medications and makes them less effective. |

| Drug | Nutrient | Interaction |
|---|---|---|
| Cholesterol Medicines (statins) | Fat Soluble Vitamins: Vitamin A, Vitamin D, Vitamin E, Vitamin K; Water Soluble Vitamins: Vitamin B12; Folic Acid CoQ10 | Bile acid sequestrants can interfere with the absorption of fats and fat-soluble vitamins. Some studies suggest that vitamin D and even iron absorption may also be adversely affected. Because of their impact on vitamin K, these drugs could cause complications in combination with blood thinners. Blood tests are advised. All vitamins should be taken at a different time from the cholesterol medicine. CoQ10 is also depleted. |
| Corticosteroids | Calcium; Vitamin D3; Potassium; Vitamin B6; Vitamin B12; Folic Acid | Cortisone-like drugs can deplete the body of vitamin D and interfere with calcium absorption and metabolism. Long term use may result in bone loss. |
| Epilepsy Drugs | Folic Acid; Vitamin B6 | Either folic acid or vitamin B6 supplements can reduce blood levels of this anticonvulsant, potentially leading to seizures. If supplementation is needed, it should be carefully monitored. |
| | Vitamin D; Calcium | Barbiturates such as phenobarbital interfere with the normal metabolism of vitamin D, and as a consequence calcium may be lost from bones. |
| Hormone Replacement Therapy | Vitamin B6; Folic acid; Vitamin E | Women using estrogen replacement therapy may need more of these vitamins. Both folic acid and B6 levels may be low, and too little vitamin B6 could be responsible for depression. |

*(continued)*

| Drug | Nutrient | Interaction |
|---|---|---|
| Iron | Calcium | Taking a calcium supplement at the same meal with an iron supplement or a multivitamin containing iron can reduce the amount of iron absorbed. To minimize interference, take these pills at different times. |
| Laxatives | Fat Soluble Vitamins: Vitamin A; Vitamin D; Vitamin D; Vitamin K | Regular use of a mineral oil laxative interferes with proper absorption of the fat-soluble vitamins. Lack of vitamin D can affect calcium and phosphate balance, and bone loss can occur. |
| Levodopa | Vitamin B6 | Vitamin B6 can reduce the effectiveness of this anti-Parkinson's disease drug. Supplementation should be avoided. |
| Tranquilizers | Riboflavin; Vitamin B 12; Vitamin C | Riboflavin and B12 may become depleted. A high dose of vitamin C may reduce the serum level of some of these drugs. |
| Potassium | Vitamin B12 | Potassium supplements can interfere with the absorption of vitamin B12. Because these medications are often taken for many weeks or months, a deficiency of this crucial vitamin could develop. Some older people may show cognitive or neurological effects of inadequate vitamin B12 even before their blood tests show a deficiency. |
| Thyroid Hormone | Iron | Iron supplements taken at the same time as thyroid replacement hormone can reduce the hormones effectiveness. Take these pills at different times. |
| | Calcium | Calcium may also interfere with levothyroxine absorption. Take these pills at least four hours apart. |

| Drug | Nutrient | Interaction |
|---|---|---|
| Ulcer Medications | Vitamin B12 | These acid suppressing drugs can reduce the absorption of vitamin B12 and is chemically bound to protein. The effect may depend upon dose and seemed to disappear after the drug is discontinued. |
| Antacids | Vitamin C; vitamins E | One theory suggests that reducing acid as effectively as these medications do could allow bacteria to survive in the stomach. These bugs may produce carcinogenic chemicals which might increase the risk of stomach or esophageal cancer. These nutrients may help protect the stomach. |
| Urinary anti-infectives | Folic Acid | Medications for urinary tract infections interfere with folic acid metabolism. Folic acid deficiencies are unusual, perhaps because the drugs are usually prescribed for less than two weeks. If used for a longer period of time, recommend supplementation. |

# FOOD AND DRUG INTERACTIONS

As healthcare practitioners we always have to be concerned with drug interactions, most often with other drugs. Considering that the average American is taking at least eight or more medications, this is a very real concern. However, drug effectiveness and possible side-effects can also be affected by foods that we eat.

While not likely being a deadly combination, foods can certainly have an impact on the medications your patients are taking. This can be manifest in one or more of several ways:

- Food may cause your medication to be absorbed less efficiently, so it becomes less effective.
- The medication might take a long period of time to get to the site of action, thus possibly creating a gap in its full potency.
- The medication's effect may be enhanced by certain foods.
- Sometimes the combination of food and medication can increase the levels of the medication in the blood.

The following list will give you a general listing of some of the food-drug interactions that you might encounter clinically. Some of these effects might dose-related so while a small dosage might not create an interaction, a higher dose might. Be sure to consult with a patient's primary care physician if there is any question as to what you are recommending.

| Drug | Food | Interaction |
|---|---|---|
| Acetaminophen | Alcohol | Both can damage the liver so all drinking of alcohol should be avoided when taking acetaminophen. |
| | Citrus fruits and Vitamin C | Can increase the side-effects and toxicity of acetaminophen. |
| | Oatmeal/high-fiber cereal | Slows down the absorption of acetaminophen. Separate ingestion by 2 hours. |
| | Echinacea | Boosts the immune system; can inflame the liver. |
| ADHD drugs | Fruit juice | May alter stomach acids leading to changes in absorption rate. |
| | Vitamin C | Similar to above. |
| | Coffee, tea, soda, chocolate | Anything with caffeine in it can speed up the heart. |
| | Ma Huang | Found in OTC diet pills-speeds up the heart and raises blood pressure. |
| Aspirin | Alcohol | Both can increase GI permeability and cause leaky gut syndrome. |
| | Ginger/ Garlic | Both are excellent blood thinners. |
| | White willow tea | The original aspirin and both blood thinners. |
| | Green tea | Same as above |
| | Iron supplements | Hard on the GI tract. |
| Allergy medicine (oral) | Alcohol | Can cause drowsiness |
| | Grapefruit juice | May cause heart problems |

*(continued)*

| Drug | Food | Interaction |
|---|---|---|
| Anticoagulants | Salads and greens | Contain Vitamin K which can increase clotting. |
| | Feverfew | Blood thinner- additive effect |
| | Garlic, Ginger, Tumeric, Ginko Biloba, Saw Palmetto | May increase bleeding |
| | Onions | More than a few ounces increase Warfarin levels |
| | Excessive supplements | More than 400IU of vitamin E and 10,000IU of vitamin A per day can thin the blood. |
| | Citrus juice or vitamin C | Can reduce the absorption of blood thinners |
| | Green tea or Matcha tea | Increases the effect of blood thinners |
| | Grapefruit juice | Can increase the level of blood thinners |
| | Soy milk | May increase bleeding |
| | Avocados | May reduce the effect of blood thinners |
| | Enzyme CoQ10 | May slightly reduce the effect of blood thinners |
| | St. John's Wort | Reduces the effectiveness of blood thinners |
| Bone-building drugs (bisphosphonates) | Calcium supplements | May affect absorption of these drugs |
| | Iron supplements | Same as above |
| | Antacids | Affects absorption; separate by 2 hours |

| Drug | Food | Interaction |
|---|---|---|
| Anxiety medicine | Alcohol | Increases the sedative and intoxicating effects; NO alcohol is recommended |
| | Coffee, tea, soda | Anything containing caffeine will work against the medication |
| | Kava, Hops, Valerian root, passionflower herb | Natural sedatives- will enhance the effect |
| | St. John's Wort | May increase the side-effects |
| | Nicotine products | May speed up elimination of the drug; reducing effectiveness |
| Arthritis medication | Alcohol | Increase risk of GI bleed or liver damage |
| | Ginger/Garlic | Can thin the blood and increase risk of bleeding |
| | Dairy | Increased stomach discomfort |
| | Panax ginseng, red clover, white willow, ginger, ginko biloba | A combination of any of these herbs can create a blood thinning effect |
| Thyroid medication | Tofu or soy products | Affect thyroid hormone production |
| | Broccoli, cauliflower, Brussels sprouts, turnips | Lower levels of circulating of thyroid hormone |
| | Dairy or Calcium supplements | Interferes with absorption of thyroid medication |
| | Oatmeal, cereal, high-fiber supplements and foods | Reduces effect of medication |
| | Stinging nettle | Nourishes the thyroid, so may need less medication |
| | All foods | Take on an empty stomach |

*(continued)*

| Drug | Food | Interaction |
|---|---|---|
| Acid blockers/ Antacids | Alcohol<br>Cranberry juice<br><br>St. John's wort<br>Spicy food, garlic, onions<br>Fast food, greasy food, sugary desserts<br>Feverfew<br>Coffee; nicotine | Stomach irritant<br>Enhances the effect of the medication<br>Increases sensitivity to sunlight<br>Tend to upset the stomach, so eat less or none of these<br>Strip the gut of healthy enzymes and beneficial flora<br>Increases risk of GI bleeding<br>Increases risk of reflux; irritates lining of stomach |
| Anti-diabetic drugs | Potatoes; starchy foods<br>Aloe vera juice<br>Alcohol<br>Potatoes, white bread, refined sugar<br>Diuretics<br>Diet pills; appetite suppressants<br>Fiber supplements | Increases blood sugar levels<br>Lowers blood sugar levels<br>Lowers blood sugar levels<br>Increases the body's need for insulin<br>Includes many herbs<br>Excite the heart, lower blood sugar levels<br>separate from these drugs |
| Anti-depressants | Coffee, tea, soda<br><br>Alcohol<br>Food | Any caffeinated beverages can increase side effects<br>Suppresses brain chemicals<br>Anti-depressants can cause weight gain |
| Urinary Incontinence Medications | Grapefruit/juice<br><br>Garlic; melatonin<br>Alcohol<br><br>Allergy medication<br><br>Potassium supplements<br><br>Diuretics<br>Coffee; tea; soda | Can increase effectiveness causing more side effects<br>Can increase side effects<br>Increases urinary frequency; increases drowsiness<br>Increases side effects including blurred vision<br>Increase likelihood of GI erosion<br>Increases urinary outflow<br>Increases urinary outflow; limit to one cup per day |

| Drug | Food | Interaction |
|---|---|---|
| Quinolone antibiotics | Dairy | Contain calcium which binds to the medication and reduces effectiveness |
| | Multivitamins | Can contain minerals which bind to the medication and reduces effectiveness |
| | Antacids | Can contain aluminum and magnesium which bind to the medication and reduce effectiveness |
| | Iron supplements | Can attach to the medication and reduce effectiveness |
| | Zinc | Same as above |
| | Birth control pills | Make birth control less effective |
| | Coffee, tea, soda | Increases side effects |
| Anti-convulsive medications | Alcohol | Interferes with the medication making it less effective |
| | Borage oil; evening primrose oil | Might cause an increase likelihood of seizures |
| | Bananas, rice | These foods can be constipating, as do anti-convulsive medications |
| | Valerian root | Can have an additive effect |
| | Grapefruit juice | Increase negative side effects |
| | Fiber supplements | Can reduce effectiveness of these medications |

(*continued*)

| Drug | Food | Interaction |
|---|---|---|
| MAO Inhibitors | St. John's Wort | Can have an additive effect; do not use within 2 weeks of medication use |
| | Antidepressants | Additive effect of increased serotonin levels |
| | Ginseng | Can cause insomnia, headaches, tremors, etc. |
| | Alcohol | Can cause an unsafe rise in blood pressure |
| | Cough syrup | Can cause an unsafe level of serotonin |
| | Cheese | Similar to alcohol reaction |
| | Eye drops; nasal sprays | Tetrahydrozoline can create hypertension reaction |
| | Coffee; tea; soda (caffeine); diet pills | Spikes blood pressure |
| Breathing medications (bronchodilators) | Caffeine | Increase heart rate |
| | Ma Huang; panax ginseng; ephedra; licorice root | All are stimulants and can have an additive effect |
| | Grilled meat | Barbeque meat releases chemicals that keep the liver from breaking down and eliminating the drug. |
| | Sugary desserts | With albuterol, increases blood sugar. |
| | Cough and cold medicines | If containing decongestants, might overstimulate the heart. |
| | Hawthorne; motherwort herb | May increase cardiac side effects |
| | Fiber; bran cereals | Separate from breathing medications by at least 2 hours |

| Drug | Food | Interaction |
|---|---|---|
| Diuretics | Bananas; asparagus; squash; green leafy vegetables; orange juice | All are rich in potassium, which may potentiate the medication |
| | Salt substitutes | Can cause potassium overload |
| | MSG | If sensitive to this, then diuretics can increase this |
| | Stinging nettle herb/tea | These remove potassium from the body |
| | Dandelion | May be a dangerous increase in potassium levels |
| Digoxin | Oatmeal or bran cereal | Slows down the breakdown of the drug- lengthening exposure time |
| | Calcium | Excessive supplementation can lead to digoxin overdose |
| | St. John's Wort | Reduces digoxin levels |
| Beta-blockers | Potassium supplements | Can cause an increase in complications |
| | Alcohol | Might slow heart rate |
| | Animal products | May increase levels of drug |
| | Albuterol | Beta-blockers may prevent your inhaler from working |
| Pain Relievers | Alcohol | When combined with pain killers, can slow down or stop the heart |
| | Kava | A natural herb used as a muscle relaxant; the sedative effect can be additive |
| | Bananas, rice or constipating foods | Painkillers are also constipating |
| | Sedating herbs | Many sedating herbs can slow down the heart |
| | Potatoes and apples | Contain pectin, which slows the heart rate |
| | Smoking | Reduces the effect of painkillers due to speeding elimination of the drug |



(*continued*)

| Drug | Food | Interaction |
|---|---|---|
| Statins | Alcohol<br><br>Grapefruit juice | Alcohol damages the liver, which is where statins work<br>Spikes the blood level of statins and increases side effects |
| Lithium | Table salt<br><br><br><br>Coffee; tea; soda; chocolate | Too little salt can decrease lithium levels in the blood; too much can increase levels-both dangerous<br>Can reduce serum levels of lithium |
| Nitrates | Alcohol<br>Arginine supplements or sexual enhancement supplements<br>Nicotine products | Can lower blood pressure<br>Can lead to a low blood pressure via vasodilation<br><br>Lowers the effect of nitrate medication |
| Sleeping medication | Alcohol<br><br>GABA supplements<br><br>Sedative herbs<br><br>Coffee; black tea | Can cause a fatal reduction in heart rate and breathing<br>Similar actions can have an additive effect<br>Similar actions can have an additive effect<br>Nullifies the effect of the medication |
| Oral contraceptives | Vitamin A<br>Coffee; tea; soda; chocolate<br>Diet pills; appetite suppressants; energy drinks<br>Grapefruit juice<br><br><br>Chasteberry; black cohosh; licorice; motherwort; saw palmetto; wild yam | Increases levels of vitamin A<br>Hormones increase the effect of caffeine<br>Can be stimulants and cause the same problems as above<br><br>Can significantly raise the levels of estradiol levels- a hormone<br>Work on the same hormonal system as this medication |

| Drug | Food | Interaction |
|---|---|---|
| Erectile dysfunction medications | Grapefruit juice; pomegranate juice | Seem to increase blood levels of these medications |
| | Alcohol | Can mimic the same side effects as these medications |
| | Hawthorne; devil's claw; mist etoe; fenugreek; figwort; Sheperd's purse; digitalis leaf; motherwort | All these herbs affect the heart |

# NUTRIENT-NUTRIENT INTERACTIONS

When we think of pharmaceutical actions, we are confident that each individual drug targets a specific or similar site of action. There can be interactions between drugs but each drug is given for a specific purpose and most other drugs are designed to counteract side effects.

When considering a nutritional supplement or a given food, there are numerous vitamins and minerals involved and they usually interact with each other. As stated previously, we don't eat a particular food just because it has one nutrient in it. All foods have a varied complex of vitamins, minerals and other substances that make the effective as fuel for our bodies.

This chapter is designed to give you a review of some of the interactions between nutrients and what nutrients might affect others. It is for this reason that it is always recommended that a properly blended full spectrum multiple formula offers the best option for patients.

| Nutrient | Nutrient | Interaction |
|---|---|---|
| Vitamin A | Calcium | Excessive vitamin A might affect calcium absorption |
| Vitamin D | Calcium | Vitamin D improves calcium absorption |
| Zinc | Copper | Excessive zinc depletes copper |
| Vitamin A | Zinc | Zinc transports vitamin A |
| Vitamin C | Selenium | Selenium makes vitamin C more bioavailable |
| Vitamin E | Vitamin C | Increases antioxidant properties |
| Calcium | Magnesium | Opposite effects on nerves |
| Magnesium | Vitamin D | Magnesium converts vitamin D into its active form to help with calcium absorption |

## POSITIVE AND NEGATIVE INTERACTIONS BETWEEN THE COMPONENTS VITAMIN-MINERAL COMPLEXES

| Micronutrient | Interactions with another vitamin or mineral | The nature of interaction |
|---|---|---|
| Vitamin A | Vitamins E, C | Protects vitamin A from oxidation |
| | Zinc | Required for metabolism of vitamin A and its transformation into active form |
| Vitamin $B_1$ | Vitamin $B_6$ | Slows transformation of vitamin $B_1$ into biologically active form |
| | Vitamin $B_{12}$ | Enhances allergic reaction to vitamin $B_1$. Cobalt ion in the molecule of cyanocobalamin contributes to destruction of vitamin $B_1$ |
| Vitamin $B_6$ | Vitamin $B_{12}$ | Cobalt ion in the molecule of cyanocobalamin contributes to destruction vitamin $B_6$ |
| Vitamin $B_9$ | Zinc | Inhibits the absorption of vitamin $B_9$ due to formation of insoluble complexes |
| | Vitamin C | Promotes conservation of vitamin $B_9$ in tissues |
| Vitamin $B_{12}$ | Vitamins C, $B_1$; iron, copper | Under the action of vitamins C, $B_1$, iron and copper, vitamin $B_{12}$ is turned to useless analogs |
| Vitamin E | Vitamin C | Restores oxidized vitamin E |
| | Selenium | Strengthens antioxidant effects of each other |
| Iron | Calcium, zinc | Reduces the absorption of iron |
| | Vitamin A | Increases the absorption of iron. The level of hemoglobin in case of joint admission of iron and vitamin A is higher than when taking only iron |

*(continued)*

| Micronutrient | Interactions with another vitamin or mineral | The nature of interaction |
|---|---|---|
| Iron (*con't*) | Vitamin C | Increases the absorption of iron, enhances iron absorption in the gastrointestinal tract |
| Calcium | Vitamin D | Increases bioavailability of calcium, potentiates calcium absorption in bone tissue |
| | Magnesium | Reduces absorption of calcium |
| | Zinc | Reduces absorption of calcium |
| Magnesium | Vitamin $B_6$ | Promotes absorption of magnesium, penetration and retention of magnesium in the cells |
| | Calcium | Reduces the absorption of magnesium |
| Manganese | Calcium, iron | Impairs absorption of manganese |
| Copper | Zinc | Reduces the absorption of copper |
| Molybdenum | Copper | Reduces absorption of molybdenum |
| Chrome | Iron | Reduces absorption of chromium |
| Zinc | Vitamin $B_9$ (Folic acid) | Inhibits the absorption of zinc due to the formation of insoluble complexes |
| | Calcium, iron, copper | Reduces absorption of zinc in the intestine |
| | Vitamin $B_2$ | Increases the bioavailability of zinc |

# COMMON MEDICATIONS AND OCULAR SIDE EFFECTS

It should be obvious to eyecare professionals to realize that the eyes are an integral part of the human body. Whatever we eat or ingest in any way affects all the parts of our body, including our eyes. This is especially true of medications.

The following table lists some of the more common medications taken for a number of different physical conditions. Included in the table are the brand name and generic name of each medication, as well as what it is used for and how it affects the eyes. Some of these medications may have variations and updated formulas on the market. Therefore, please have patients check with their physician before taking any medication so that you are aware of any possible visual side effects.

| COMMON MEDICATIONS AND THEIR OCULAR SIDE EFFECTS | | | |
|---|---|---|---|
| **Brand Name** | **Generic Name** | **Indications** | **Ocular Side Effects** |
| Accutane | Isotretinoin | Difficult cases of cystic acne; keratinization disorders; folliculitis; psoriasis. | Redness, dry eyes, corneal opacities, tearing, optic neuritis, dryness, light sensitivity, floaters, contact lens intolerance, night blindness. |
| Achromycin | Tetracycline | Acne; chlamydia. | Retinal hemorrhage, decreased vision, headaches, light sensitivity, nearsightedness, enlarged blind spot. |

(continued)

| COMMON MEDICATIONS AND THEIR OCULAR SIDE EFFECTS (*con't*) | | | |
|---|---|---|---|
| **Brand Name** | **Generic Name** | **Indications** | **Ocular Side Effects** |
| Actifed | Pseudoephedrine | Allergic rhinitis; allergic conjunctivitis and skin manifestations; motion sickness. | Hallucinations, decreased eye pressure, dilated pupils, dry eyes. |
| Adipex | Phentermine | Weight control. | Decreased vision, headache, cataracts, hallucinations, double vision, disturbed accommodation. |
| Aricept | Donepezil | Alzheimer's Disease | Cataracts, glaucoma, retinal hemorrhages, conjunctival hemorrhages, eye irritation. blepharitis, dry eyes, floaters. |
| Arimidex | Anastrozole | Breast cancer | Cataracts |
| Atrovent | Ipratropium bromide | Rhinitis. | Worsened narrow-angle glaucoma, pink eye, dry eyes, blurred vision, pain. |
| Benadryl | Diphenhydramine | Allergic rhinitis; allergic conjunctivitis and skin manifestations; motion sickness. | Visual-field constriction, hallucinations, retinal hemorrhage. |
| Betoptic | Betaxolol | Open-angle glaucoma. | Hallucinations, decreased tear flow, redness, double vision, drooping eyelids. |
| Cafergot | Ergotamine | Migraines. | Spasming and constriction of blood vessels in all parts of the eye. |
| Cardizem | Diltiazem | Angina due to coronary-artery spasm; mild to moderate hypertension. | Pain, redness, dizziness, hallucinations, tearing, irritation, |

| Brand Name | Generic Name | Indications | Ocular Side Effects |
|---|---|---|---|
| Catapres | Clonidine | Hypertension. | Eye irritation, dry eyes, hallucinations, dilated pupils. |
| Celebrex | Celecoxib | Anti-inflammatory | Visual field defects, blurred vision |
| Coumadin | Warfarin sodium | Venous thrombosis; atrial fibrillation with embolization; pulmonary emboli; coronary occlusion. | Tearing, cataracts, hemorrhage, decreased vision, yellowing of eyes. |
| Desyrel | Trazodone | Depression. | Optic neuritis, lazy eye, retinal or subconjunctival hemorrhage, light sensitivity, dry eyes, decreased vision. |
| Detrol | Tolterodine tartrate | Bladder control. | Headaches, dryness, blurred near vision. |
| Diabinese | Chlorpropamide | Diabetes. | Optic neuritis, disturbed color vision, retinal hemorrhage, light sensitivity, double vision. |
| Dilantin | Phenytoin | Epilepsy. | Retinal hemorrhage, nystagmus, yellowing of eyes, double vision, disturbed accommodation, flashing lights, glare sensitivity, disturbed color vision. |
| Dimetapp | Brompheniramine | Coughs and upper respiratory symptoms, including nasal congestion, associated with allergy or common cold. | Different-sized pupils, visual-field constriction, hallucinations, dryness, double vision. |
| Diuril | Chlorothiazide | Hypertension; edema associated with congestive heart failure, cirrhosis, or corticosteroid or estrogen therapy. | Edema, retinal hemorrhage, disturbed accommodation, nearsightedness, yellow vision. |

*(continued)*

| COMMON MEDICATIONS AND THEIR OCULAR SIDE EFFECTS (*con't*) | | | |
|---|---|---|---|
| **Brand Name** | **Generic Name** | **Indications** | **Ocular Side Effects** |
| Donnatal | Phenobarbital | Epilepsy; anxiety. | Blind spots, hallucinations, lazy eye, optic neuritis, involuntary eye movements, blurred vision, pupil dilation |
| Elavil | Amitriptyline | Depression. | Hallucinations, retinal hemorrhage, lazy eye, optic neuritis, dry eyes, yellowing, increased eye pressure. |
| Enduron | Methyclothiazide | Hypertension; edema associated with congestive heart failure, cirrhosis, premenstrual tension, or corticosteroid or estrogen therapy. | Edema, retinal hemorrhage, decreased vision, disturbed accommodation, redness, light sensitivity. |
| Fosamax | Alendronate Sodium | Osteoporosis | Inflammation of the sclera, uveitis |
| Humulin | Insulin | Diabetes. | Decreased pupil reaction, double vision, involuntary eye movements, blurred vision. |
| Imitrex | Sumatriptan | Migraines | Eye muscle weakness, accommodative disorder, dilated pupils, ocular hemorrhage, eye pain, conjunctivitis, ocular edema, corneal opacities |
| Inderal | Propranolol | Hypertension. | Drooping eyelids, double vision, decreased vision, hallucinations, dry eyes, headache. |
| Ismelin | Guanethidine | Hypertension. | Light sensitivity, burning, double vision, accommodative spasm, flashing lights. |
| Lamictal | Lomtrigine | Seizures | Dizziness, ataxia, sedation, involuntary eye movements, blurred vision, double vision. |

## COMMON MEDICATIONS AND OCULAR SIDE EFFECTS

| Brand Name | Generic Name | Indications | Ocular Side Effects |
|---|---|---|---|
| Lanoxin | Digoxin | Congestive heart failure; atrial fibrillation or flutter; atrial tachycardia. | Optic neuritis, disturbed color vision, blurred vision, headache, yellow vision, hallucinations, glare sensitivity, halos around lights, double vision. |
| Lasix | Furosemide | Hypertension, Diuretic | Blurred vision, dizziness, headache |
| Librium | Chlordiazepoxide | Anxiety | Disturbed depth perception, retinal hemorrhage, disturbed accommodation, yellowing of eye. |
| Lipitor | Atorvastatin | Cholesterol control | Swelling around eyelids, red eyes, itching, myasthenia gravis, headaches, light sensitivity. |
| Lithobid | Lithium | Manic phase of bipolar disorder | Blind spots, retinal or subconjunctival hemorrhage, hallucinations, light sensitivity, involuntary eye movements, dry eyes. |
| Mellaril | Thioridazine | Psychosis. | Night blindness, blind spots, cataracts, blurred vision, hallucinations, lazy eye, crossed eyes, light sensitivity, yellowing, optic atrophy, discolored eyes. |
| Mevacor | Lovastatin | Elevated cholesterol. | Cataracts, blurred vision, headache. |
| Motrin | Ibuprofen | Osteoarthritis; pain; fever. | Blind spots, visual field constriction, lazy eye, retinal hemorrhage, optic neuritis, dry eyes. |
| Niaspan | Niacin | Elevated cholesterol | Blurred vision, toxic lazy eye, central blind spot, glaucoma, protruding eyes. |

*(continued)*

| COMMON MEDICATIONS AND THEIR OCULAR SIDE EFFECTS (*con't*) | | | |
|---|---|---|---|
| **Brand Name** | **Generic Name** | **Indications** | **Ocular Side Effects** |
| Norpramin | Desipramine | Depression | Hallucinations, lazy eye, optic neuritis, dryness, blurred vision, headache, light sensitivity, yellowing, disturbed accommodation. |
| Norvasc | Amlodipine | Hypertension, angina | Blurred vision, headache, vertigo, visual distortion, yellowing. |
| Ortho-Novum | Norethindrone | Birth control | Optic neuritis, blind spots, halos around lights, cataracts, headache, yellowing of eyes. |
| Orudis | Ketoprofen | Rheumatoid arthritis. | Decreased vision, retinal or subconjunctival hemorrhage, eye pain, hallucinations, visual field constriction, pink eye. |
| Paxil | Paroxetine hydrochloride | Depression | Dry eyes, abnormal vision, blurred vision, headache, dizziness. |
| Pepcid | Famotidine | Duodenal ulcer; benign gastric ulcer. | Decreased vision, hallucinations, retinal or subconjunctival hemorrhage, light sensitivity, yellowing. |
| Plaquenil | Hydroxychloro-quine | Malaria; rheumatoid arthritis; lupus erythematosus | Cataracts, eye pigmentation, focusing difficulty, eye blisters, eye muscle paralysis, accommodative difficulty, halos around lights, hallucinations, night blindness, flashing lights. |
| Pravachol | Pravastatin sodium | Cholesterol control | Headache, muscle weakness, dizziness. |
| Premarin | Estrogen | Menopause; osteoporosis; female hypogonadism; atrophic vaginitis; breast cancer; prostate cancer | Optic neuritis, blind spots, disturbed color vision, yellowing of eyes, myopia, dry eyes, fluctuations in vision, contact lens intolerance. |

## COMMON MEDICATIONS AND OCULAR SIDE EFFECTS

| Brand Name | Generic Name | Indications | Ocular Side Effects |
|---|---|---|---|
| Prozac | Fluoxetine | Depression. | Pain, light sensitivity, dry eye, iritis, cataracts, double vision, drooping eyelids. |
| Restoril | Temazepam | Insomnia; anxiety, tension, agitation; skeletal-muscle spasms | Pain, disturbed accommodation, yellowing, hallucinations, tearing, burning, light sensitivity, nystagmus. |
| Retin-A | Tretinoin | Acne | Skin dryness, light sensitivity red eyes, red eyelids. |
| Ritalin | Methylpheni-date | Attention deficit hyperactivity disorder | Retinal or subconjunctival hemorrhage, dilated pupils, hallucinations, blurred vision, redness. |
| Rogaine | Minoxidil | Hair re-growth | Increased eye pressure, decreased vision, optic neuritis, blurred vision. |
| Synthroid | Levothyroxine | Hypothyroidism | Decreased vision, double vision, drooping eyelids, yellow eyes, dry eyes. |
| Tagamet | Cimetidine | Ulcers | Hallucinations, light sensitivity, blurred vision, redness, irritation/dryness. |
| Tavist | Clemastine | Mild allergy symptoms | Decreased vision, dryness, light sensitivity, eyelid swelling, hallucinations, different-sized pupils. |
| Tenormin | Atenolol | Hypertension (beta-blocker) | Decreased vision, hallucinations, dryness, burning, redness, yellow eyes. |
| Timoptic | Timolol maleate | Glaucoma | Dryness, burning, blurred vision, pupil size variations droopy eyelids, nearsightedness, hallucinations. |
| Topamax | Topiramate | Anti-seizure | Glaucoma, increase tearing, double vision, myopia |

*(continued)*

| COMMON MEDICATIONS AND THEIR OCULAR SIDE EFFECTS (*con't*) | | | |
|---|---|---|---|
| **Brand Name** | **Generic Name** | **Indications** | **Ocular Side Effects** |
| Tylenol | Acetaminophen | Fever; mild pain | Hallucinations, disturbed color vision, double vision, redness. |
| Viagra | Sildenafil | Erectile Dysfunction | Blurred vision, yellow vision, sensitivity to light, blue vision, double vision, hemorrhages, burning. |
| Voltaren | Diclofenac | Rheumatoid arthritis; osteoarthritis; post-eye surgery | Blurred vision, night blindness, lazy eye, blind spots, bleeding in the eye, itching, tearing, light sensitivity. |
| Xanax | Alprazolam | Anxiety; depression | Disturbed color vision, disturbed accommodation, pain, hallucinations, uncontrolled eye movements, yellowing. |
| Zestril | Ace-Inhibitor | Hypertension | Yellow eyes, dizziness, headache. |
| Zantac | Ranitidine | Gastric ulcers | Disturbed color vision, hallucinations, blurred vision, eyelid swelling, yellowing, redness. |
| Zocor | Simvastatin | Elevated cholesterol | Blurred vision, worsened cataracts, eye muscle weakness. |
| Zoloft | Sertaline | Anti-depressant | Eye pain, blind spots, dry eyes, light sensitivity, double vision, increase tearing. |
| Zyrtec | Cetirizine | Allergies | Ocular melanoma, glaucoma, ocular hemorrhage, loss of accommodation, dryness, headache, loss of visual field. |

# THE NEED FOR SUPPLEMENTS

A BASIC QUESTION WE MUST ASK IS: "DO WE NEED TO USE NUTRITIONAL supplements or just recommend a new diet for patients?" While we'd like to think that we can get all of our proper nutrition from our dietary intake, it's not that simple. Even the general supermarket has "artificial" foods and poor nutrient-dense foods that lack the basic nutrients that we need daily. And then there are the "junk" or packaged foods that contain artificial ingredients that our bodies do not even recognize. It seems amazing that there is a "health-food" section the market. Isn't that redundant? So, yes, we need to supplement our diets. Even the American Medical Association now recommends a full spectrum vitamin/mineral supplement for most individuals, especially if you are over the age of 50.

Taking full-spectrum supplements, eating clean (meaning almost no junk food) and exercise is the best investment you can make in both short and long-term health. Overworked soils, cold storage, food processing, and over-cooking strips today's foods of a large amount of their nutritional value. Therefore, nutritional needs have overtaken the number of micronutrients provided in the very best of daily diets.

A high-quality multivitamin/mineral supplement should be the foundation for every nutrition program. Despite all of the studies proving the efficacy of multiple supplements in preventing disease and promoting optimal health, too many physicians still don't take them seriously because they are too busy to read micronutrient studies published in nutrition and biochemistry journals. A large amount of published scientific evidence suggests a full-spectrum multivitamin/mineral supplement is good insurance, and would markedly improve health, e.g. degenerative diseases of the eye, heart disease, cancer, and immune function, particularly for those who consume inadequate diets, which is the majority of people in the U.S. The chart below is data collected by the USDA that compares nutrition intake vs. recommendations from 1970, as compared to 2018. While overall consumption increased in most categories, the consumption continues to be below the daily recommendations. It speaks volumes about the need for a daily multiple supplement.

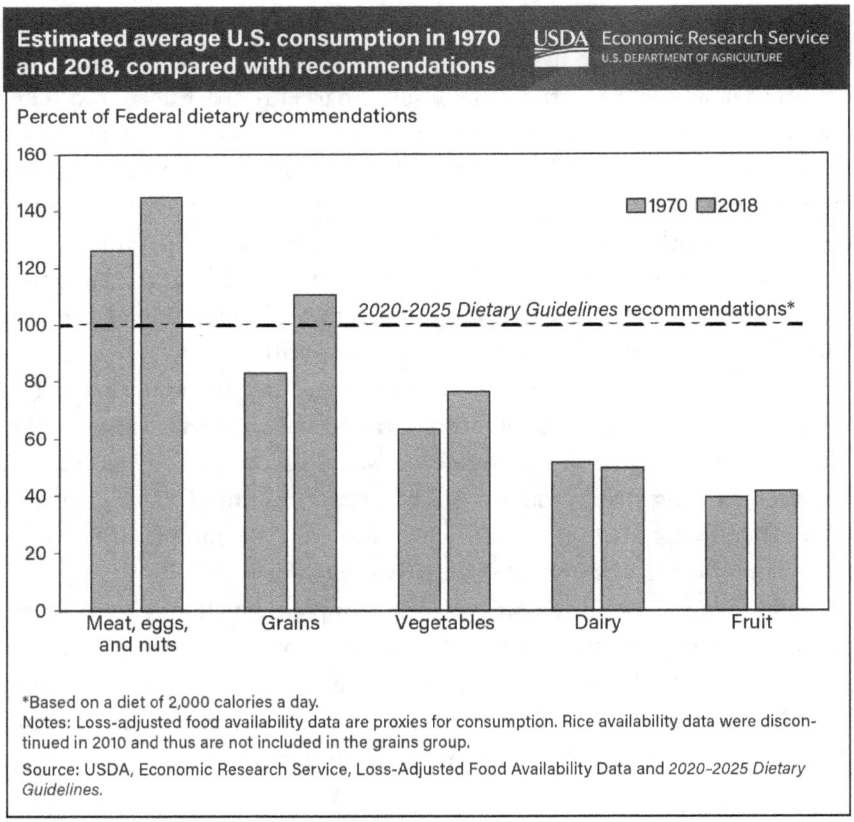


**Figure 7.** Estimated average US consumption of foods

## RDA VS. NUTRITION REQUIREMENTS

The Food and Nutrition Board at the National Academy of Science sets the Recommended Daily Allowances (RDA) or Daily Values at minimal levels needed to prevent diseases like scurvy and rickets, not at levels reflecting nutrition science that supports optimal health. Optimal health is desired by today's baby boom aging population, most of which are determined to maintain health and vitality through the aging process. Unfortunately, most supplement consumers notice very little difference in their health, their wellbeing, or their energy level when taking inexpensive low-potency one-a-day formulations that only include the suggested RDA amounts of the most basic vitamins and minerals.

Our bodies are made up of about 100 trillion cells. Each cell derives nutrients from foods and supplements, which are carried to them via the bloodstream. The semi-permeable membrane that surrounds each cell only allows a select number of micronutrients to cross its barrier. Minerals are especially subject to this regulatory process and cross the cells membrane based on our body's bioelectrical needs at any given time.

Each nutrient we consume must compete for transport space, as well as space within the cell. Therefore, long-term consumption of excessively high amounts of any single nutrient causes a deficiency of another nutrient. For the most part, our bodies are well equipped to handle nutrients in excess– they simple excrete them as waste material. However, nutrient deficiencies caused by poor diets or excessive supplementation of single nutrients cannot be compensated for. If there is not enough of a given nutrient crossing the cell membrane, the cell cannot make that up that deficiency by any other means. The concept of ratios tells us that all nutrients need to be present and available to our cells and they need to be present in relative potencies based on their bioelectrical potential.

There are four general misconceptions regarding vitamins and minerals for patient care:

1. *They are completely safe*—While that is mostly true, they can be abused and cause dangerous effects if not taken appropriately, just like any over-the-counter item.
2. *They are ineffective*—The effectiveness of nutrients is much more subtle and long-term than it is with drugs, but they are effective nevertheless.
3. *They are all the same*—Not true, especially when a multiple vitamin is considered. The type, form, and amount of each nutrient can make a major difference in how it works.
4. *More is better*—This is the most common misconception; just because a certain amount is effective, it does not mean that ten times that amount is ten times more effective!

To successfully evaluate patients for nutrient deficiencies, it would be helpful to assess their nutrient intake. That sounds like a daunting task and one best left for nutritionists. However, you can usually get a good sense of their basic diet by asking just a few general questions:

1. How many servings of fruits and vegetables do you eat on a daily basis? (Note: one serving is a ¼ cup or a "handful"). Also be aware that people will ALWAYS over-estimate this amount, and by the way, French fries do NOT count as a vegetable serving! The CDC recommends 9-13 servings per day!
2. How many times a week do you eat fish (and what kind)? We now realize that smaller, fatty fish (sardines, mackerel, anchovies, herring, salmon, etc.) at least three times a week are the best for Omega-3 intake.
3. Do you eat baked goods? These contain simple sugars and "bad" carbs, which is worse than eating "bad" cholesterol! Substituting good carbohydrates in vegetables is better.

4. Do you take a full spectrum multiple vitamin/mineral supplement? While we think that eating a "balanced" diet should supply an adequate vitamin intake, it rarely happens so a supplement is usually required. Also, a few pills will not overcome a bad diet!

5. Do you limit the portion of food that you eat at each meal? Most people eat until the plate or box is empty. Limiting portions can allow you to eat better, more nutrient-dense foods while still losing weight.

## HOW TO CHOOSE HIGH QUALITY MULTIPLE SUPPLEMENTS

Given the national state of optometric licensing, just about every optometrist is allowed to order blood panels. An exact review of vitamin levels in the blood will offer an excellent roadmap of how to proceed in making the appropriate recommendations to your patients. However, knowing a bit of the science and how nutrients are used in supplement form would be helpful. For example, it is often overlooked that there are eight different

| FDA-regulated products | Pre-market approval | Pre-market notification | Labeling | Mandatory adverse event reporting | GMPs | Facility registration | Advertising (FTC or FDA) |
|---|---|---|---|---|---|---|---|
| Foods | | ✓ | ✓ | | ✓ | ✓ | ✓ |
| Dietary supplements | | ✓ | ✓ | ✓ | ✓ | ✓ | ✓ |
| Drugs | ✓ | | ✓ | ✓ | ✓ | ✓ | ✓ |

**Figure 8:** FDA Regulation for Consumed Products

forms of vitamin E and almost all supplements use the tocopherol form and not the tocotrienol form, which has many benefits. Also, vitamin D should be in the D3 form, not D2, which is one-third as effective. Good basic information can be reviewed at the National Institutes of Health, Office of Dietary Supplements website. (https://ods.od.nih.gov/)

So, what should be considered in a vitamin supplement to help eye health? There are literally dozens of companies in the US alone making hundreds of different products in this category. Patients don't want to be taking handfuls of pills so try to get as much nutrition as you can in fewer pills. The products should have a valid scientific rationale available for anyone to review, as well as a website that puts science first before price and marketing. Any company that promotes making "millions of dollars" on selling their products should be looked at with suspect. Health goals should be directed toward patient well-being; the income will follow.

The first thing the practitioner should look for is a product that is a good blend and balance of nutrients that is formulated around the very latest science in nutritional medicine. This is going to take a bit of time considering the number of companies and products that are out there. And it's unlikely that the practitioner is going to become a biochemist in the process. Make sure that the scientific rationale for their ingredients is available (usually on their website).

One thing to consider is the form of the pill being offered. Hard-pressed pills are typically found to not break down effectively in the body. A capsule or gel-cap is preferable. Liquids are also an effective way to get nutritional supplements absorbed.

A full-spectrum supplement should be designed to slow the progression of chronic degenerative disease, including all eye diseases. There should be efficacious amounts of properly balanced fat-soluble vitamins, particularly as it relates to the latest vitamin A and vitamin D research. Vitamin A should be in the retinol form, not beta-carotene. It should contain potent amounts of the full-spectrum of B vitamins for the proper maintenance of homocysteine, specifically B6, B12 and folic acid. There should also be 400 IUs of the complete spectrum of Vitamin E with a balanced mixture of both natural d-alpha tocopherol (not the synthetic form of "dl-alpha tocopherol") and mixed tocopherol oils containing gamma and delta tocopherols and tocotrienols.

Supplemental iron has been linked to heart disease, so it should be iron-free for men and post-menopausal women. It should also contain the full army of "job-specific" antioxidants that both prevent free-radical damage, as well as neutralize the effects of previous oxidative damage. In addition, there should be efficacious amounts of eye-specific carotenoids: lutein esters (not free lutein) and pure zeaxanthin, to assure proper xanthophyll transport to the retina. Meso-zeaxanthin is not needed in a supplement because it is formed from lutein in the visual cycle. And it should also contain the spectrum of minerals in their most bioavailable form to ensure proper cellular bioelectrical and enzymatic response. For example, zinc oxide (found in AREDS formulas) is the poorest absorbable form of zinc!

Speaking of AREDS, while it has become the "gold standard" for AMD therapy, the study did not show efficacy in the early stages of the disease (only slowed progression from stage 3 to 4). It is better to recommend a full-spectrum supplement to support overall health.

Office protocols for approaching the patient should be done in a caring manner. First, diagnose the condition and carefully explain the options to the patient. Then, hand the patient a brochure that fully explains the recommended product. If they decide to purchase it right away, take the bottle to the front desk to dispense as a convenience to the patient. If they want to consider it later, simply let your office staff know (via a routing slip) that the product was discussed with the patient. They can again ask the patient if they wish to make the purchase at the initial visit or at a later time. Either way, the patient knows that it is available and something that can assist in their treatment. A two-week follow up phone call asking about the status of the nutrient recommendation can increase compliance by up to 50% in many cases. This also demonstrates the doctor's commitment to the welfare of the patient.

Learning about nutrition can be a life-long proposition but can be extremely beneficial to you and your patients. While we are not biochemists or nutritionists, we should learn some of the basics of nutrition to make intelligent decisions about what to recommend to our patients. If we don't, someone else will.

There are many practices that follow the medical model and bill for most of their services. Technically, nutritional supplements are not allowed as a tax deduction since they are OTC and are most often taken for general health purposes. However, the IRS has published this section in their "Publication 502": *"You cannot include in medical expenses the cost of nutritional supplements, vitamins, herbal supplements, "natural medicines," etc. unless they are recommended by a medical practitioner as treatment for a specific medical condition diagnosed by a physician. Otherwise, these items are taken to maintain your ordinary good health, and are not for medical care."* These rules apply to Flexible Spending Accounts (FSA) and Health Savings Accounts (HAS) accounts. Thus, if you are making a specific recommendation of a nutritional product for dry eyes, the cost of that supplement may be eligible as a tax deduction. This will obviously facilitate the purchase if someone is cautious about their insurance not covering the product. Be sure the patient confirms that this is true for their particular situation with their tax consultant.

There are several outlets for learning about general nutrition and ocular nutrition. The most efficient start would be to log into the Ocular Wellness and Nutrition Society (OWNS) www.ocularnutritionsociety.org). This non-profit organization was started in 2008 by the author with a board of directors who exhibited high professional standards and education about nutrition and its role in ocular health. The society offers several avenues to education on ocular health including a Fellowship certification, and is currently instigating a program of ocular nutrition electives in all of the optometry schools around the country. Optometry students are eligible for free membership and the educational opportunities are top quality.

Also, consider the American Nutrition Association (ANA) (www.theana.org). The ANA champions the science and practice of personalized nutrition. Nutrition science and scientific integrity support the ANA's work and mission and must always be upheld in relationships with the corporate sector. The ANA is committed to its values first and foremost and does not compromise these for financial gain or any other purposes. They offer a peer-reviewed that curates and disseminates original research in nutrition to empower researchers and healthcare professionals. They also offer a Certified Personalized Nutrition Practitioner certification program.

The area of nutritional support for eye health is rapidly growing and emerging science is showing more and more benefits for patients to take a nutritional supplement. However, just taking a few vitamins won't overcome a poor diet. We need to support our patients in turning around their lifestyle to assure that they not only see better into their later years but that their "health-span" is almost as long as their "life-span". With the proper counseling from their primary eyecare practitioner, our patients can see clearly throughout their entire lifetime.

# CONCLUSION

Optometrists are primary care providers. This is not only true for eye health, but we are very often the ones on the front lines of human health and disease. Many first-year students might be thinking the same way I did prior to my acceptance to optometry school: "How can I spend four years just studying eyes?" It didn't take me long to realize that the eyes "are a part of the body", and, in many cases, indicators of our general health. Aside from the obvious physical diseases that are evident while looking at the eyes and visual system (affected by hypertension, diabetes, MS, etc.), there can be many other subtle health disorders that we can forestall with appropriate action.

It is true that "we are what we eat" because diet is such a large part of our lifestyle that it can alter our biochemistry much quicker than alterations in our genetic makeup. Nutrition courses are just beginning to be accepted into the medical school curriculum but as of now, less than 10 percent of medical education is devoted to nutrition. The numbers are even worse lower for optometric education.

The reason for this book is to provide eyecare practitioners scientific and unbiased information on the role of that nutrition plays in eye health and disease. It is my hope that this volume will provide a spark for you to learn more about the role of nutrition in eye and overall health. As I have said, as optometrists, just because we focus on the eyes, doesn't mean we should be blind to the influence of less obvious factors that we don't see.

# REFERENCES


## PART 1:
### Digestion, Absorption, Metabolism

Dunne LJ, Kirschmann JD, Nutrition Search, Inc. Nutrition Almanac. 3rd ed. McGraw-Hill; 1990.

Balch JF, Balch PA. Prescription for Nutritional Healing. Avery Publishing 1990, Garden City New York

Kutsky RJ. Handbook of Vitamins, Minerals and Hormones Van Nostrand Reinhold Company, New York, 1981

### Micronutrients—Vitamins

Aaraj S, Kausar A, Khan SA. Vitamin D deficiency: A risk factor for myopia in children—a cross sectional study in a tertiary care centre. J Pak Med Assoc. 2022 Jun;72(6):1075-1079.

Age-Related Eye Disease Study Research Group. A randomized, placebo-controlled, clinical trial of high-dose supplementation with vitamins C and E and beta carotene for age-related cataract and vision loss: AREDS report no. 9. Arch Ophthalmol 2001;119:1439-52.

Bailey LB, Caudill MA. Folate. In: Erdman JW, Macdonald IA, Zeisel SH, eds. Present Knowledge in Nutrition. 10th ed. Washington, DC: Wiley-Blackwell; 2012:321-42.

Blaner WS. Vitamin A and Provitamin A Carotenoids. In: Marriott BP, Birt DF, Stallings VA, Yates AA, eds. Present Knowledge in Nutrition. 11th ed. Cambridge, Massachusetts: Wiley-Blackwell; 2020:73-91.

Carr AC, Frei B. Toward a new recommended dietary allowance for vitamin C based on antioxidant and health effects in humans. Am J Clin Nutr 1999;69:1086-107.

Chin KY, Pang KL, Soelaiman IN. Tocotrienol and Its Role in Chronic Diseases. Adv Exp Med Biol. 2016;928:97-130.

Deng H, Chen Y, Xing J, et al. Systematic low-grade chronic inflammation and intrinsic mechanisms in polycystic ovary syndrome. Front Immunol. 2024 Dec 19;15:1470283.

## REFERENCES


Ellison DL, Moran HR. Vitamin D: Vitamin or Hormone? Nurs Clin North Am. 2021 Mar;56(1):47-57.

Gaul C, Diener HC, Danesch U; Migravent® Study Group. Improvement of migraine symptoms with a proprietary supplement containing riboflavin, magnesium and Q10: a randomized, placebo-controlled, double-blind, multicenter trial. J Headache Pain. 2015;16:516.

Haghdoost F, Togha M. Migraine management: Non-pharmacological points for patients and health care professionals. Open Med (Wars). 2022 Nov 23;17(1):1869-1882.

Hui F, Tang J, Williams PA, et al Improvement in inner retinal function in glaucoma with nicotinamide (vitamin B3) supplementation: A crossover randomized clinical trial. Clin Exp Ophthalmol. 2020 Sep;48(7):903-914

Institute of Medicine. Food and Nutrition Board. Dietary Reference Intakes: Thiamin, Riboflavin, Niacin, Vitamin B6, Folate, Vitamin B12, Pantothenic Acid, Biotin, and Choline. Washington, DC: National Academy Press; 1998.

Jacob RA, Sotoudeh G. Vitamin C function and status in chronic disease. Nutr Clin Care 2002;5:66-74.

Lane B. Nutrition and Vision, 273-274 in Bland J, Ed. 1984-85 Yearbook of Nutritional Medicine New Canaan, CT: Keats, 1985

Kirschmann, John D. Nutrition Almanac 6th Edition N/A Nutrition Search, Inc Published: December 21, 2006

Murkey SP, Agarwal A, Pandit P, Kumar S, Jaiswal A. Unveiling the Spectrum of Ophthalmic Manifestations in Nutritional Deficiencies: A Comprehensive Review. Cureus. 2023 Dec 11;15(12):e50311.

Namazi N, Heshmati J, Tarighat-Esfanjani A. Supplementation with Riboflavin (Vitamin B2) for Migraine Prophylaxis in Adults and Children: A Review. Int J Vitam Nutr Res. 2015;85(1-2):79-87.

Pang KL, Chin KY. The Role of Tocotrienol in Protecting Against Metabolic Diseases. Molecules. 2019 Mar 6;24(5):923.

Ross A. Vitamin A. In: Ross AC, Caballero B, Cousins RJ, Tucker KL, Ziegler TR, eds. Modern Nutrition in Health and Disease. 11th ed. Baltimore, MD: Lippincott Williams & Wilkins; 2014:260-77.

Rautiainen S, Lindblad BE, Morgenstern R, Wolk A. Vitamin C supplements and the risk of age-related cataract: a population-based prospective cohort study in women. Am J Clin Nutr. 2010 Feb;91(2):487-93

Sen CK, Khanna S, Roy S. Tocotrienols: Vitamin E beyond tocopherols. Life Sci. 2006 Mar 27;78(18):2088-98.

Sperduto RD, Hu TS, Milton RC, et al. The Linxian cataract studies. Two nutrition intervention trials. Arch Ophthalmol 1993;111:1246-53.

Tripkovic L, Lambert H, Hart K, et al. Comparison of vitamin D2 and vitamin D3 supplementation in raising serum 25-hydroxyvitamin D status: a systematic review and meta-analysis. Am J Clin Nutr. 2012 Jun;95(6):1357-64.

Ureña Torres PA, Souberbielle JC, Solal MC. Bone Fragility in Chronic Kidney Disease Stage 3 to 5: The Use of Vitamin D Supplementation. Metabolites. 2022 Mar 20;12(3):266.

## Micronutrients—Minerals

Lane, B.C. (1981). Calcium, Chromium, Protein, Sugar and Accommodation in Myopia. In: Fledelius, H.C., Alsbirk, P.H., Goldschmidt, E. (eds) Third International Conference on Myopia Copenhagen, August 24–27, 1980. Documenta Ophthalmologica Proceedings Series, vol 28. Springer, Dordrecht.

Li SO, Wang JL, Bjørklund G, et al. Serum copper and zinc levels in individuals with autism spectrum disorders. Neuroreport. 2014 Oct 22;25(15):1216-20.

## Other Helpful Nutrients (carotenoids)

Backhouse, S, Gentle, A. Scleral remodeling in myopia and its manipulation: a review of recent advances in scleral strengthening and myopia control. *Annals of Eye Science* 2018; 3:5 (21 January 2018).

Canovai A, Tribble JR, Jöe M, et al Pyrroloquinoline quinone drives ATP synthesis in vitro and in vivo and provides retinal ganglion cell neuroprotection. Acta Neuropathol Commun. 2023 Sep 8;11(1):146

Eggersdorfer M, Wyss A. Carotenoids in human nutrition and health. Arch Biochem Biophys. 2018 Aug 15.652:18-26.

Goralczyk R. Beta-carotene and lung cancer in smokers: review of hypotheses and status of research. Nutr Cancer. 2009;61(6):767-74.

Karns, K. Herr, AE. Human Tear Protein Analysis Enabled by an Alkaline Microfluidic Homogeneous Immunoassay *Analytical Chemistry* 2011 *83* (21), 8115-8122

Lançon A, Frazzi R, Latruffe N. Anti-Oxidant, Anti-Inflammatory and Anti-Angiogenic Properties of Resveratrol in Ocular Diseases. *Molecules*. 2016 Mar 2;21(3):304.

Liu Y, Gan L, Zhao B, Yu K, Wang Y, Männistö S, Weinstein SJ, Huang J, Albanes D. Untargeted metabolomic profiling identifies serum metabolites associated with type 2 diabetes in a cross-sectional study of the Alpha-Tocopherol, Beta-Carotene Cancer Prevention (ATBC) Study. Am J Physiol Endocrinol Metab. 2023 Feb 1;324(2):E167-E175.

Manabe K, Kaidzu S, Tsutsui A, et al. Effects of French maritime pine bark/bilberry fruit extracts on intraocular pressure for primary open-angle glaucoma. *J Clin Biochem Nutr*. 2021 Jan;68(1):67-72

Murienne BJ, Chen ML, Quigley HA, Nguyen TD. The contribution of glycosaminoglycans to the mechanical behaviour of the posterior human sclera. J R Soc Interface. 2016 Jun;13(119):20160367

Olk RJ, Peralta E, Gierhart DL, et al. (2017) Combination Therapy with Dietary Zeaxanthin for Neovascular Age-Related Macular Degeneration. A Randomized Clinical Trial. *J Clin Exp Ophthalmol* 8: 692.

Olk JR, Peralta E, Gierhart DL, et al. Triple combination therapy and zeaxanthin for the treatment of neovascular age- related macular degeneration: an interventional comparative study and cost- effectiveness analysis. *Int J Ret Vitreous.* 2015;1:22.

Omenn GS, Goodman G, Thornquist M, Grizzle J, Rosenstock L, Barnhart S, Balmes J, Cherniack MG, Cullen MR, Glass A, et al. The beta-carotene and retinol efficacy trial (CARET) for chemoprevention of lung cancer in high-risk populations: smokers and asbestos-exposed workers. Cancer Res. 1994 Apr 1;54(7 Suppl):2038s-2043s.

Ranard KM, Jeon S, Mohn ES, et al. Dietary guidance for lutein: consideration for intake recommendations is scientifically supported. *Eur J Nutr.* 2017 Dec;56 (Suppl 3):37-42.

Richer SP, Cebold B, Katkar M, et al. Restoration of Central Macular Pigment Dip with Dietary RR Zeaxanthin Supplementation in Patients with AMD. Adv *Ophthalmol Vis Syst.* 7(3): 00219

Richer S, Patel S, Sockanathan S, Ulanski LJ 2nd, Miller L, Podella C. Resveratrol based oral nutritional supplement produces long-term beneficial effects on structure and visual function in human patients. Nutrients. 2014 Oct 17;6(10):4404-20.

Richer S, Stiles W, Ulanski L, Carroll D, Podella C. Observation of human retinal remodeling in octogenarians with a resveratrol based nutritional supplement. Nutrients. 2013 Jun 4;5(6):1989-2005.

Shyam R, Vachali P, Gorusupudi A, et al. All three human scavenger receptor class B proteins can bind and transport all three macular xanthophyll carotenoids. *Arch Biochem Biophys.* 2017 Nov 15;634:21-28

Shyam R, Gorusupudi A, Nelson K, et al. RPE65 has an additional function as the lutein to meso-zeaxanthin isomerase in the vertebrate eye. *Proc Natl Acad Sci U S A.* 2017 Oct 10;114(41):10882-10887

Steigerwalt, Robert Jr, et. Effects of Mirtogenol on ocular blood flow and intraocular hypertension in asymptomatic subjects *Molecular Vision* 2008; 14:1288-1292

Wu J, Cho E, Willett WC, Sastry SM, Schaumberg DA. Intakes of Lutein, Zeaxanthin, and Other Carotenoids and Age-Related Macular Degeneration During 2 Decades of Prospective Follow-up. JAMA Ophthalmol. 2015 Dec;133(12):1415-24.

## Eye Structures and Supportive Nutrients

### *Herbal Therapy*

Abdi F, Alimoradi Z, Haqi P, et al. Effects of phytoestrogens on bone mineral density during the menopause transition: a systematic review of randomized, controlled trials. Climacteric. 2016;19(6):535-545.

Al-Khamees, W. A. A.; Schwartz, M. D.; Alrashdi, S.; Algren, A. D.; Morgan, B. W. (2011). "Status Epilepticus Associated with Borage Oil Ingestion". Journal of Medical Toxicology. 7 (2): 154–157.

Algranti E, Mendonça EM, Ali SA, Kokron CM, Raile V. Occupational asthma caused by Ipe (Tabebuia spp) dust. J Investig Allergol Clin Immunol 2005;15:81-3.

Anheyer D, Lauche R, Schumann D, et al. Herbal medicines in children with attention deficit hyperactivity disorder (ADHD): a systematic review. Complementary Therapies in Medicine. 2017;30:14-23.

Asher GN, Corbett AH, Hawke RL. Common herbal dietary supplement-drug interactions. American Family Physician. 2017;96(2):101-107.

"Assessment report on Euphrasia officinalis L. and Euphrasia rostkoviana Hayne, herba (Page 13)" (PDF). Archived from the original (PDF) on 2018-06-18. Retrieved 2017-03-29.

Calvo MI, Cavero RY. Medicinal plants used for ophthalmological problems in Navarra (Spain). J Ethnopharmacol. 2016 Aug 22;190:212-8.

Chan SW, Tomlinson B. Effects of bilberry supplementation on metabolic and cardiovascular disease risk. Molecules. 2020;25(7):1653.

Comfrey". Drugs.com. 17 July 2017. Retrieved 22 May 2018.

de Oliveira JR, Camargo SEA, de Oliveira LD. Rosmarinus officinalis L. (rosemary) as therapeutic and prophylactic agent. J Biomed Sci. 2019 Jan 9;26(1):5.

Dodson, Craig D.; Stermitz, Frank R. (1986). "Pyrrolizidine alkaloids from borage (Borago officinalis) seeds and flowers". Journal of Natural Products. 49 (4): 727–728.

Farnsworth, N. R. Alfalfa pills and autoimmune diseases. Am J Clin Nutr. 1995;62:1026-1028.

Fern, Ken (30 July 2021). "Useful Tropical Plants Smilax officinalis". tropical.theferns.info. Tropical Plants Database. Retrieved 20 March 2022.

Final report on the safety assessment of Calendula officinalis extract and Calendula officinalis. Int J Toxicol. 2001;20 Suppl 2:13-20.

Freye E, GLeske J. Siberian ginseng results in beneficial effects on glucose metabolism in diabetes type 2 patients: a double blind placebo-controlled study in comparison to panax ginseng. Int J Clin Nutr. 2013;1:11-17.

Genus: Myrica L. Germplasm Resources Information Network. United States Department of Agriculture. 2006-12-14. Retrieved 2010-10-31.

Ghasemzadeh Rahbardar M, Hosseinzadeh H. Therapeutic effects of rosemary (Rosmarinus officinalis L.) and its active constituents on nervous system disorders. Iran J Basic Med Sci. 2020 Sep;23(9):1100-1112.

Ghazanfarpour M, Sadeghi R, Roudsari RL, et al. Red clover for treatment of hot flashes and menopausal symptoms: a systematic review and meta-analysis. Journal of Obstetrics and Gynaecology. 2016;36(3):301-311.

Ginkgo. Natural Medicines website. Accessed at naturalmedicines.therapeuticresearch.com on March 9, 2020. [Database subscription].

Gleason, Henry A. and Arthur Cronquist. 1991. "Manual of Vascular Plants of Northeastern United States and Adjacent Canada, Second Edition." The New York Botanical Garden. Bronx, New York.

Goldenseal. Natural Medicines website. Accessed at naturalmedicines.therapeuticresearch.com on December 23, 2019. [Database subscription].

## REFERENCES


Grčević M, Kralik Z, Kralik G, Galović O. Effects of dietary marigold extract on lutein content, yolk color and fatty acid profile of omega-3 eggs. J Sci Food Agric. 2019 Mar 30;99(5):2292-2299.

Grieve, Maud (1971). A Modern Herbal: The Medicinal, Culinary, Cosmetic and Economic Properties, Cultivation and Folk-lore of Herbs, Grasses, Fungi, Shrubs, & Trees with All Their Modern Scientific Uses, Volume 1. Courier Corporation. p. 292. ISBN 9780486227986.

Herbert, V. and Kasdan, T. S. Alfalfa, vitamin E, and autoimmune disorders. Am J Clin Nutr 1994;60:639-640.

Holubarsch CJF, Colucci WS, Meinertz T, et al. The efficacy and safety of Crataegus extract WS 1442 in patients with heart failure: the SPICE trial. European Journal of Heart Failure. 2008;10(12):1255-1263.

Holubarsch CJF, Colucci WS, Eha J. Benefit-risk assessment of Crataegus extract US 1442: an evidence-based review. American Journal of Cardiovascular Drugs. 2018;18(1):25-36.

Howard, Michael (1987): Traditional Folk Remedies. Century. p.136

Jurzysta, M. and Waller, G. R. Antifungal and hemolytic activity of aerial parts of alfalfa (Medicago) species in relation to saponin composition. Adv. Exp Med Biol 1996;404:565-574.

Kanadys W, Baranska A, Jedrych M, et al. Effects of red clover (Trifolium pratense) isoflavones on the lipid profile of perimenopausal and postmenopausal women—A systematic review and meta-analysis. Maturitas. 2020;132:7-16.

Kang JM, Lin S. Ginkgo biloba and its potential role in glaucoma. Current Opinion in Ophthalmology. 2018;29(2):116-120.

Kast, RE (2001). "Borage oil reduction of rheumatoid arthritis activity may be mediated by increased cAMP that suppresses tumor necrosis factor-alpha". International Immunopharmacology. 1 (12): 2197–9.

Koch E, Busse WR, Juretzek W, et al. Hawthorn. In: Coates PM, Betz JM, Blackman MR, et al., eds. Encyclopedia of Dietary Supplements. 2nd ed. New York, NY: Informa Healthcare; 2010:411-422.

Malinow, M. R., Connor, W. E., McLaughlin, P., et al. Cholesterol and bile acid balance in Macaca fascicularis. Effects of alfalfa saponins. J Clin Invest 1981;67:156-162.

Malinow, M. R., McLaughlin, P., and Stafford, C. Alfalfa seeds: effects on cholesterol metabolism. Experientia 5-15-1980;36:562-564.

Mármol I, Sánchez-de-Diego C, Jiménez-Moreno N, Ancín-Azpilicueta C, Rodríguez-Yoldi MJ. Therapeutic applications of rose hips from different Rosa species. Int J Mol Sci. 2017;18:1137

McClure C, Bollen M, Buttolph L, et al. Safety and tolerability of Pau d' Arco (Tabebuia avellanedae) for primary dysmenorrhea: A single-arm, open-label trial on adults ages 18-45. Adv Integr Med 2022;9:159-166.

## REFERENCES

McKenna DJ, Plotnikoff GA. Goldenseal. In: Coates PM, Betz JM, Blackman MR, et al., eds. Encyclopedia of Dietary Supplements. 2nd ed. New York, NY: Informa Healthcare; 2010:379-390.

Mei, Nan; Guo, Lei; Fu, Peter P.; Fuscoe, James C.; Luan, Yang; Chen, Tao (October 2010). "Metabolism, genotoxicity, and carcinogenicity of Comfrey". Journal of Toxicology and Environmental Health Part B: Critical Reviews. 13 (7–8): 509–526.

Miroddi M, Calapai G, Navarra M, et al. Passiflora incarnata L: ethnopharmacology, clinical application, safety and evaluation of clinical trials. Journal of Ethnopharmacology. 2013;150(3):791-804.

Myrica L. Plants of the World Online. Board of Trustees of the Royal Botanic Gardens, Kew. 2017. Retrieved 9 July 2020.

Naghibi Harat, Z.; Kamalinejad, M.; Sadeghi, M. R.; Sadeghipour, H. R.; Eshraghian, M. R. (2009-05-10). "A Review on Ruta graveolens L. Its Usage in Traditional Medicine and Modern Research Data". Journal of Medicinal Plants. 8 (30): 1–19.

Nguyen JT, Tian D-D, Tanna RS, et al. Assessing transporter-mediated natural product-drug interactions via in vitro-in vivo extrapolation: clinical evaluation with a probe cocktail. Clinical Pharmacology and Therapeutics. November 11, 2020.

Oh E, Kim Y, Park SY, et al. The fruit of Acanthopanax senticosus Harms improves arterial stiffness and blood pressure: a randomized, placebo-controlled trial. Nutr Res Pract. 2020;14:322-333.

Parandin R, Ghowsi M, Dadbod A. Protective effects of hydroalcoholic extract of Rosa canina L. fruit on cyclophosphamide-induced testicular toxicity in mice. Avicenna J Phytomed 2023;13:7-17. View abstract.

Phetcharat L, Wongsuphasawat K, Winther K. The effectiveness of a standardized rose hip powder, containing seeds and shells of Rosa canina, on cell longevity, skin wrinkles, moisture, and elasticity. Clin Interv Aging. 2015;10:1849-56.

Quidel Kramer F, Ortigoza Á. Ginkgo biloba for the treatment of tinnitus. Medwave. 2018;18(6):e7295.

"Smilax officinalis Kunth". Plants of the World Online. Royal Botanic Gardens, Kew. Retrieved 20 March 2022.

Srinivasan, S. R., Patton, D., Radhakrishnamurthy, B., et al. Lipid changes in atherosclerotic aortas of Macaca fascicularis after various regression regimens. Atherosclerosis 1980;37:591-601.

Strømgaard K, Vogensen SB, Steet J, et al. Ginkgo. In: Coates PM, Betz JM, Blackman MR, et al., eds. Encyclopedia of Dietary Supplements, 2nd ed. New York, NY: Informa Healthcare; 2010:332-338.

Swain E, Li CP, Poulton JE (April 1992). "Development of the Potential for Cyanogenesis in Maturing Black Cherry (Prunus serotina Ehrh.) Fruits". Plant Physiology. 98 (4): 1423–1428.

Tohda C, Matsui M, Inada Y, et al. Combined Treatment with Two Water Extracts of Eleutherococcus senticosus Leaf and Rhizome of Drynaria fortunei Enhances

Cognitive Function: A Placebo-Controlled, Randomized, Double-Blind Study in Healthy Adults. Nutrients. 2020 Jan 23;12. pii: E303.

Vaneková Z, Rollinger JM. Bilberries: curative and miraculous—a review on bioactive constituents and clinical research. Frontiers in Pharmacology. 2022;13:909914.

Wallace ED, Oberlies NH, Cech NB, et al. Detection of adulteration in Hydrastis canadensis (goldenseal) dietary supplements via untargeted mass spectrometry-based metabolomics. Food and Chemical Toxicology. 2018;120:439-447

Werbach MR, Murray MT. Botanical Influences on Illness. Tarzana, CA. Third Line Press, 1994

Yemm RS, Poulton JE (June 1986). "Isolation and characterization of multiple forms of mandelonitrile lyase from mature black cherry (Prunus serotina Ehrh.) seeds". Archives of Biochemistry and Biophysics. 247 (2): 440–5.

Zhang L, Hasegawa I, Ohta T. Anti-inflammatory cyclopentene derivatives from the inner bark of Tabebuia avellanedae. Fitoterapia 2016;109:217-23.

# PART II: Eye Disorders

## Accommodative Insufficiency/spasm:

Bharadwaj SR, Ravisankar C, Roy S, Satgunam P. Fluctuations of Steady-State Accommodation Is a Marker for Screening Spasm of Near Reflex. Transl Vis Sci Technol. 2021 Sep 1;10(11):9.

Bharadwaj SR, Roy S, Satgunam P. Spasm of Near Reflex: Objective Assessment of the Near-Triad. Invest Ophthalmol Vis Sci. 2020 Jul 1;61(8):18.

Lindberg L. Akkommodaatiospasmi [Spasm of accommodation]. Duodecim. 2014;130(2):168-73. Finnish. PMID: 24605432.

Manna P, Karmakar S, Bhardwaj GK, Mondal A. Accommodative spasm and its different treatment approaches: A systematic review. Eur J Ophthalmol. 2023 May;33(3):1273-1286.

## Arcus Senilis

Ang M, Wong W, Park J, et al. Corneal arcus is a sign of cardiovascular disease, even in low-risk persons. Am J Ophthalmol. 2011 Nov;152(5):864-71.e1.

Barchiesi BJ, Eckel RH, Ellis PP. The cornea and disorders of lipid metabolism. Surv Ophthalmol. 1991 Jul-Aug;36(1):1-22.

François J, Feher J. Arcus senilis. Doc Ophthalmol. 1973 Feb 21;34(1):165-82.

Rohrbach JM, Lisch W, Seitz B. The cornea as an indicator for systemic diseases. Hautarzt. 2019 May;70(5):371-382.

Vurgese S, Panda-Jonas S, Saini N, et al. Corneal arcus and its associations with ocular and general parameters: the Central India Eye and Medical Study. Invest Ophthalmol Vis Sci. 2011 Dec 20;52(13):9636-43.

## Blepharitis

Bernardes TF, Bonfioli AA. Blepharitis. Semin Ophthalmol. 2010 May;25(3):79-83.

Bron AJ, Tiffany JM, Gouveia SM, Yokoi N, Voon LW. Functional aspects of the tear film lipid layer. Exp Eye Res. 2004;78:347–360

Bron AJ, Tiffany JM. The contribution of meibomian disease to dry eye. Ocul Surf. 2004;2:149–165

Duke-Elder S, Wybar KC. The Anatomy of the Visual System. London: Henry Kimpton; 1961:577

Foulks GN, Bron AJ. Meibomian gland dysfunction: a clinical scheme for description, diagnosis, classification, and grading. Ocul Surf. 2003;1:107–126

Gilbard JP. Dry eye, blepharitis and chronic eye irritation: divide and conquer. J Ophthalmic Nurs Technol. 1999 May-Jun;18(3):109-15.

Jackson WB. Blepharitis: current strategies for diagnosis and management. Can J Ophthalmol. 2008 Apr;43(2):170-9.

Korb DR, Henriquez AS. Meibomian gland dysfunction and contact lens intolerance. J Am Optom Assoc. 1980;51:243–251

## Blepharospasm

Coscarelli JM. Essential blepharospasm. Semin Ophthalmol. 2010 May;25(3):104-8.

Defazio G, Hallett M, Jinnah HA, Conte A, Berardelli A. Blepharospasm 40 years later. Mov Disord. 2017 Apr;32(4):498-509.

Hassell TJW, Charles D. Treatment of Blepharospasm and Oromandibular Dystonia with Botulinum Toxins. Toxins (Basel). 2020 Apr 22;12(4):269.

Serefoglu Cabuk K, Tunc U, Ozturk Karabulut G, et al Serum calcium, magnesium, phosphorus, and vitamin D in benign essential blepharospasm. Graefes Arch Clin Exp Ophthalmol. 2020 Jun;258(6):1293-1297.

## Cataracts

Abdelkader H, Alany RG, Pierscionek B. Age-related cataract and drug therapy: opportunities and challenges for topical antioxidant delivery to the lens. J Pharm Pharmacol. 2015 Apr;67(4):537-50.

Ang MJ, Afshari NA. Cataract and systemic disease: A review. Clin Exp Ophthalmol. 2021 Mar;49(2):118-127.

Babizhayev MA, Yegorov YE. Telomere Attrition in Human Lens Epithelial Cells Associated with Oxidative Stress Provide a New Therapeutic Target for the Treatment, Dissolving and Prevention of Cataract with N-Acetylcarnosine Lubricant Eye Drops. Recent Pat Drug Deliv Formul. 2016;10(2):82-129.

Braakhuis AJ, Donaldson CI, Lim JC, Donaldson PJ. Nutritional Strategies to Prevent Lens Cataract: Current Status and Future Strategies. Nutrients. 2019 May 27;11(5):1186.

Bunce GE. Nutrition and cataract. Nutr Rev. 1979 Nov;37(11):337-43.

Hodge WG, Whitcher JP, Satariano W. Risk factors for age-related cataracts. Epidemiol Rev. 1995;17(2):336-46.

James M, Crabbe C, Harding JJ. Diabetic and galactosaemic cataracts. Trans Ophthalmol Soc U K (1962). 1982;102 Pt 3:342-5.

Jiang, Hong et al. Dietary vitamin and carotenoid intake and risk of age-related cataract The American Journal of Clinical Nutrition, Volume 109, Issue 1, 43 – 54

Lim JC, Caballero Arredondo M, Braakhuis AJ, Donaldson PJ. Vitamin C and the Lens: New Insights into Delaying the Onset of Cataract. Nutrients. 2020 Oct 14;12(10):3142.

Wu SY, Leske MC. Antioxidants and cataract formation: a summary review. Int Ophthalmol Clin. 2000 Fall;40(4):71-81.

Wang L, Li X, Men X, et al. Research progress on antioxidants and protein aggregation inhibitors in cataract prevention and therapy (Review). Mol Med Rep. 2025 Jan;31(1):22.

Zhao L, Chen XJ, Zhu J, et al Lanosterol reverses protein aggregation in cataracts. Nature. 2015 Jul 30;523(7562):607-11. Erratum in: Nature. 2015 Oct 22;526(7574):595.

## Computer Vision Syndrome (Digital Eyestrain)

Cao Y, Yang L, Qiao X, et al. J. Dietary astaxanthin: an excellent carotenoid with multiple health benefits. Crit Rev Food Sci Nutr. 2023;63(18):3019-3045.

Lem DW, Gierhart DL, Davey PG. Can Nutrition Play a Role in Ameliorating Digital Eye Strain? Nutrients. 2022 Sep 27;14(19):4005.

Lie I., Watten R.G. VDT work, oculomotor strain, and subjective complaints: An experimental and clinical study. Ergonomics. 1994;37:1419–1433

Luberto F., Gobba F., Broglia A. Temporary myopia and subjective symptoms in video display terminal operators. Med. Lav. 1989;80:155–163. - PubMed

Nishida Y, Berg PC, Shakersain B, et al. Astaxanthin: Past, Present, and Future. Mar Drugs. 2023 Sep 28;21(10):514.

Yoshida K, Sakai O, Honda T, et al. Effects of Astaxanthin, Lutein, and Zeaxanthin on Eye-Hand Coordination and Smooth-Pursuit Eye Movement after Visual Display Terminal Operation in Healthy Subjects: A Randomized, Double-Blind Placebo-Controlled Intergroup Trial. Nutrients. 2023 Mar 17;15(6):1459.

## Cornea

Gumus K. On the Horizon: Biologics and Nutrients for Neurotrophic Keratitis. Eye Contact Lens. 2021 Mar 1;47(3):154-156.

Markoulli M, Ahmad S, Arcot J, et al. TFOS Lifestyle: Impact of nutrition on the ocular surface. Ocul Surf. 2023 Jul;29:226-271.

Ruiz-Lozano RE, Hernandez-Camarena JC, Loya-Garcia D, et al. The molecular basis of neurotrophic keratopathy: Diagnostic and therapeutic implications. A review. Ocul Surf. 2021 Jan;19:224-240.

## Diabetic Retinopathy

Cheung N, Mitchell P, Wong TY. Diabetic retinopathy. Lancet. 2010 Jul 10;376(9735):124-36.

Kollias AN, Ulbig MW. Diabetic retinopathy: Early diagnosis and effective treatment. Dtsch Arztebl Int. 2010 Feb;107(5):75-83; quiz 84.

Liu J, Qin L, Zheng J, et al. Research Progress on the Relationship between Vitamins and Diabetes: Systematic Review. Int J Mol Sci. 2023 Nov 15;24(22):16371.

Roohbakhsh A, Karimi G, Iranshahi M. Carotenoids in the treatment of diabetes mellitus and its complications: A mechanistic review. Biomed Pharmacother. 2017 Jul;91:31-42.

Saxena S, Jalali S, Meredith TA, Holekamp NM, Kumar D. Management of diabetic retinopathy. Indian J Ophthalmol. 2000 Dec;48(4):321-30.

Schönlau F, Rohdewald P. Pycnogenol for diabetic retinopathy. A review. Int Ophthalmol. 2001;24(3):161-71.

Shah J, Cheong ZY, Tan B, et al. Dietary Intake and Diabetic Retinopathy: A Systematic Review of the Literature. Nutrients. 2022 Nov 25;14(23):5021.

Sluijs I, Cadier E, Beulens JW, van der A DL, Spijkerman AM, van der Schouw YT. Dietary intake of carotenoids and risk of type 2 diabetes. Nutr Metab Cardiovasc Dis. 2015 Apr;25(4):376-81.

Talegawkar S, Tobias D, Fung T, et al. Dietary Patterns and Risk of Type 2 Diabetes: A Systematic Review [Internet]. Alexandria (VA): USDA Nutrition Evidence Systematic Review; 2024 Nov

Yedjou CG, Grigsby J, Mbemi A, et al. The Management of Diabetes Mellitus Using Medicinal Plants and Vitamins. Int J Mol Sci. 2023 May 22;24(10):9085.

## Dry Eye

Bhandarkar NS, Shetty K, Narendra P, et al. Nutrition and diet for dry eye disease: Insights toward holistic management. Indian J Ophthalmol. 2024 Oct 1;72(10):1412-1423.

Cong Y, Zhang Y, Han Y, et al. Recommendations for nutritional supplements for dry eye disease: current advances. Front Pharmacol. 2024 May 30;15:1388787.

Demirci G., Karaman Erdur S., Ozsutcu M, et al. Dry Eye Assessment in Patients with Vitamin D Deficiency. Eye Contact Lens. 2018;44:S62–S65.

Hwang J.S., Lee Y.P., Shin Y.J. Vitamin D Enhances the Efficacy of Topical Artificial Tears in Patients with Dry Eye Disease. Cornea. 2019;38:304–310.

Liu A, Ji J. Omega-3 essential fatty acids therapy for dry eye syndrome: a meta-analysis of randomized controlled studies. Med Sci Monit. 2014 Sep 6;20:1583-9.

Molina-Leyva I, Molina-Leyva A, Bueno-Cavanillas A. Efficacy of nutritional supplementation with omega-3 and omega-6 fatty acids in dry eye syndrome: a systematic review of randomized clinical trials. Acta Ophthalmol. 2017 Dec;95(8):e677-e685.

Pellegrini M, Senni C, Bernabei F, et al. The Role of Nutrition and Nutritional Supplements in Ocular Surface Diseases. Nutrients. 2020 Mar 30;12(4):952.

Ponzini E, Scotti L, Grandori R, et al. Lactoferrin Concentration in Human Tears and Ocular Diseases: A Meta-Analysis. Invest Ophthalmol Vis Sci. 2020 Oct 1;61(12):9.

Rand AL, Asbell PA. Nutritional supplements for dry eye syndrome. Curr Opin Ophthalmol. 2011 Jul;22(4):279-82.

Rolando M, Barabino S. Dry Eye Disease: What Is the Role of Vitamin D? Int J Mol Sci. 2023 Jan 11;24(2):1458.

Saccà SC, Cutolo CA, Ferrari D, et al. The Eye, Oxidative Damage and Polyunsaturated Fatty Acids. Nutrients. 2018 May 24;10(6):668

Wojtowicz JC, Butovich I, Uchiyama E, Aronowicz J, Agee S, McCulley JP. Pilot, prospective, randomized, double-masked, placebo-controlled clinical trial of an omega-3 supplement for dry eye. Cornea. 2011 Mar;30(3):308-14.

Yang C.-H., Albietz J., Harkin D.G., et al. Impact of Oral Vitamin D Supplementation on the Ocular Surface in People with Dry Eye and/or Low Serum Vitamin D. Contact Lens Anterior Eye. 2018;41:69–76

Zhang Y, Lu C, Zhang J. Lactoferrin and Its Detection Methods: A Review. Nutrients. 2021 Jul 22;13(8):2492.

## Floaters

Aleman AI, Kiryakoza L, Sridhar J, Sengillo J. Management of vitreous floaters: a review. Curr Opin Ophthalmol. 2024 Sep 1;35(5):365-368.

Katsanos A, Tsaldari N, Gorgoli K, et al. Safety and Efficacy of YAG Laser Vitreolysis for the Treatment of Vitreous Floaters: An Overview. Adv Ther. 2020 Apr;37(4):1319-1327.

Milston R, Madigan MC, Sebag J. Vitreous floaters: Etiology, diagnostics, and management. Surv Ophthalmol 2016; 61:211–227.

Sendrowski DP, Bronstein MA. Current treatment for vitreous floaters. Optometry. 2010 Mar;81(3):157-61.

Vandorselaer T, Van De Velde F, Tassignon MJ. Eligibility criteria for Nd-YAG laser treatment of highly symptomatic vitreous floaters. Bull Soc Belge Ophtalmol. 2001;(280):15-9.

## Glaucoma

Aliancy, J., Stamer, W.D., Wirostko, B. A Review of Nitric Oxide for the Treatment of Glaucomatous Disease. *Ophthalmol Ther* 6, 221–232 (2017).

Asrani S, Zeimer R, Wilensky J, et al Large diurnal fluctuations in intraocular pressure are an independent risk factor in patients with glaucoma. J Glaucoma. 2000; 9:134-42

Bussel II, Aref AA. Dietary factors and the risk of glaucoma: a review. Ther Adv Chronic Dis. 2014 Jul;5(4):188-94.

Canovai A, Tribble JR, Jöe M, et al Pyrroloquinoline quinone drives ATP synthesis in vitro and in vivo and provides retinal ganglion cell neuroprotection. Acta Neuropathol Commun. 2023 Sep 8;11(1):146

## REFERENCES


Engin KN, Engin G, Kucuksahin H, et al. Clinical evaluation of the neuroprotective effect of alpha-tocopherol against glaucomatous damage. Eur J Ophthalmol. 2007 Jul-Aug;17(4):528-33

Goulart Nacácio E, Silva S, Occhiutto ML, Costa VP. The use of Nicotinamide and Nicotinamide riboside as an adjunct therapy in the treatment of glaucoma. Eur J Ophthalmol. 2023 Sep;33(5):1801-1815

Hui F, Tang J, Williams PA, et al Improvement in inner retinal function in glaucoma with nicotinamide (vitamin B3) supplementation: A crossover randomized clinical trial. Clin Exp Ophthalmol. 2020 Sep;48(7):903-914

Kutsky, RJ. Handbook of Vitamins, Minerals and Hormones (Van Nostrand Reinhold Company, New York 1981

Lee SY, Tseng VL, Kitayama K, et al. Associations Between Niacin Intake and Glaucoma in the National Health and Nutrition Examination Survey. J Glaucoma. 2023 Jun 1;32(6):443-450.

Musa, M, et al. Nutritional factors: benefits in glaucoma and ophthalmic pathologies Life. 2023;13:1120

Ohguro H, Ohguro I, Yagib S. Effects of Black Currant Anthocyanins on Intraocular Pressure in Healthy Volunteers and Patients with Glaucoma Journal of Ocular Pharmacology and Therapeutics 29(1), October 2012

Shanmugham V, Subban R. Ninety-day repeated oral toxicity study of saponified *Capsicum annum* fruit extract with 50% Capsanthin in Sprague-Dawley Rats with a 28-day recovery period. Toxicol Rep. 2022 Mar 5;9:323-336.

Shanmugham V, Subban R. Extraction of capsanthin from Capsicum annum L fruits and its effect on carbomer-induced intraocular pressure in Albino Wistar rats. J Food Biochem. 2021 Jul;45(7):e13776.

Shanmugham V, Subban R. Capsanthin from Capsicum annum fruits exerts anti-glaucoma, antioxidant, anti-inflammatory activity, and corneal pro-inflammatory cytokine gene expression in a benzalkonium chloride-induced rat dry eye model. J Food Biochem. 2022 Oct;46(10):e14352.

Swartwout, GM. Glaucoma Solutions: Prevention and Reversal. Swartwout GM. Vision for Living, 1983

Tribble JR, Otmani A, Sun S, et al. Nicotinamide provides neuroprotection in glaucoma by protecting against mitochondrial and metabolic dysfunction. Redox Biol. 2021 Jul;43:101988

Wang YE, Tseng VL, Yu F, et al. Association of Dietary Fatty Acid Intake With Glaucoma in the United States. JAMA Ophthalmol. 2018 Feb 1;136(2):141-147.

Zhang Y, Zhao Z, Ma Q, et al. Association between dietary calcium, potassium, and magnesium consumption and glaucoma PLOS ONE Published: October 18, 2023

## Grave's Disease (Thyroid Eye Disease)

Hoang TD, Stocker DJ, Chou EL, Burch HB. 2022 Update on Clinical Management of Graves Disease and Thyroid Eye Disease. Endocrinol Metab Clin North Am. 2022 Jun;51(2):287-304.

Khong JJ, McNab A. Medical treatment in thyroid eye disease in 2020. Br J Ophthalmol. 2021 Mar;105(3):299-305.

Kumari R, Chandra Saha B. Advances in the management of thyroid eye diseases: An overview. Int Ophthalmol. 2018 Oct;38(5):2247-2255.

Strianese D. Efficacy and Safety of Immunosuppressive Agents for Thyroid Eye Disease. Ophthalmic Plast Reconstr Surg. 2018 Jul/Aug;34(4S Suppl 1):S56-S59.

Weiler DL. Thyroid eye disease: a review. Clin Exp Optom. 2017 Jan;100(1):20-25.

## Headaches

Beck E. Hard-to-diagnose headache: practical tips for diagnosis and treatment. Am Fam Physician. 2013 May 15;87(10):672-3.

Dodick DW. Diagnosing Secondary and Primary Headache Disorders. Continuum (Minneap Minn). 2021 Jun 1;27(3):572-585.

Hainer BL, Matheson EM. Approach to acute headache in adults. Am Fam Physician. 2013 May 15;87(10):682-7.

Hernandez J, Molina E, Rodriguez A, et al. Headache Disorders: Differentiating Primary and Secondary Etiologies. J Integr Neurosci. 2024 Feb 20;23(2):43.

Levin M. Classification and Diagnosis of Primary Headache Disorders. Semin Neurol. 2022 Aug;42(4):406-417.

## Hordeolum (Stye)

Copeman PW. Treatment of recurrent styes. Lancet. 1958 Oct 4;2(7049):728-9.

Lindsley K, Nichols JJ, Dickersin K. Non-surgical interventions for acute internal hordeolum. Cochrane Database Syst Rev. 2017 Jan 9;1(1):CD007742.

Willmann D, Guier CP, Patel BC, Melanson SW. Hordeolum (Stye). 2024 Dec 11. In: StatPearls [Internet]. Treasure Island (FL): StatPearls Publishing; 2025 Jan–.2024 Dec 11

## Subconjunctival Hemorrhage

Hong IH, Cho BJ, Choi SH. Association between subconjunctival hemorrhage and hemorrhagic disorders: a nationwide population-based study. Sci Rep. 2023 Dec 14;13(1):22237.

Knopf HL, Carter K, Prokopius MJ. Recurrent subconjunctival hemorrhage. Compr Ophthalmol Update. 2006 May-Jun;7(3):155-6.

Mimura T, Usui T, Yamagami S, et al. Recent causes of subconjunctival hemorrhage. Ophthalmologica. 2010;224(3):133-7.

Parikh AO, Christian CW, Forbes BJ, Binenbaum G. Prevalence and Causes of Subconjunctival Hemorrhage in Children. Pediatr Emerg Care. 2022 Aug 1;38(8):e1428-e1432.

Randhawa S, Abowd M, Sharma A, Weiss JS. Anterior segment complications of a nutritional supplement. J Cataract Refract Surg. 2007 May;33(5):918-20.

Serhan HA, Alma'aitah HW, Irshaidat S, et al. Ophthalmic manifestations of nutritional deficiencies: A mini review. J Family Med Prim Care. 2022 Oct;11(10):5899-5901.

## Hypertensive Retinopathy

Cheung CY, Biousse V, Keane PA, et al. Hypertensive eye disease. Nat Rev Dis Primers. 2022 Mar 10;8(1):14.

Dziedziak J, Zaleska-Żmijewska A, Szaflik JP, et al. Impact of Arterial Hypertension on the Eye: A Review of the Pathogenesis, Diagnostic Methods, and Treatment of Hypertensive Retinopathy. Med Sci Monit. 2022 Jan 20;28:e935135.

Tsukikawa M, Stacey AW. A Review of Hypertensive Retinopathy and Chorioretinopathy. Clin Optom (Auckl). 2020 May 5;12:67-73.

Wang Z, Feng L, Wu M, et al. Hypertensive retinopathy can predict stroke: A systematic review and meta-analysis based on observational studies. J Stroke Cerebrovasc Dis. 2024 Nov;33(11):107953.

## Iritis

Doyle JO. Recurrent iritis. Br Med J. 1975 May 17;2(5967):371-2.

Fox J. Conjunctivitis, keratitis and iritis. Nursing (Lond). 1989 Nov 9-22;3(45):20-3.

Powell MA. Conjunctivitis versus iritis. J Am Acad Nurse Pract. 1990 Jul-Sep;2(3):125-6.

## Macular Degeneration

Cheung LK, Eaton A. Age-related macular degeneration. Pharmacotherapy. 2013 Aug;33(8):838-55.

Evans JR, Lawrenson JG. Antioxidant vitamin and mineral supplements for slowing the progression of age-related macular degeneration. Cochrane Database Syst Rev. 2012 Nov 14;11:CD000254.

Fursova AZh, Gesarevich OG, Gonchar AM, et al. [Dietary supplementation with bilberry extract prevents macular degeneration and cataracts in senesce-accelerated OXYS rats]. Adv Gerontol. 2005;16:76-9. Russian.

Gopinath, Bamini et al Dietary flavonoids and the prevalence and 15-y incidence of age-related macular degeneration The American Journal of Clinical Nutrition, Volume 108, Issue 2, 381 - 387

Hammond BR Jr, Johnson EJ, Russell RM, et al. Dietary modification of human macular pigment density. Invest Ophthalmol Vis Sci. 1997 Aug;38(9):1795-801.

Hobbs RP, Bernstein PS. Nutrient Supplementation for Age-related Macular Degeneration, Cataract, and Dry Eye. J Ophthalmic Vis Res. 2014 Oct-Dec;9(4):487-93.

Jiang H, Shi X, Fan Y, et al. Dietary omega-3 polyunsaturated fatty acids and fish intake and risk of age-related macular degeneration. Clin Nutr. 2021 Dec;40(12):5662-5673.

Johnson, Elizabeth J et al. Potential role of dietary n-3 fatty acids in the prevention of dementia and macular degeneration The American Journal of Clinical Nutrition, Volume 83, Issue 6, 1494S - 1498S

Landrum JT, Bone RA, Joa H, Kilburn MD, Moore LL, Sprague KE. A one-year study of the macular pigment: the effect of 140 days of a lutein supplement. Exp Eye Res. 1997 Jul;65(1):57-62.

Richer S, Stiles W, Statkute L, et al. Double-masked, placebo-controlled, randomized trial of lutein and antioxidant supplementation in the intervention of atrophic age-related macular degeneration: the Veterans LAST study (Lutein Antioxidant Supplementation Trial). Optometry. 2004 Apr;75(4):216-30.

Roy S, Khanna S, Alessio HM, Vider J, Bagchi D, Bagchi M, Sen CK. Anti-angiogenic property of edible berries. Free Radic Res. 2002 Sep;36(9):1023-31.

SanGiovanni JP, Chew EY, Clemons TE, et al. Age-Related Eye Disease Study Research Group; The relationship of dietary carotenoid and vitamin A, E, and C intake with age-related macular degeneration in a case-control study: AREDS Report No. 22. Arch Ophthalmol. 2007 Sep;125(9):1225-32.

Seddon JM, Ajani UA, Sperduto RD, et al. Dietary carotenoids, vitamins A, C, and E, and advanced age-related macular degeneration. Eye Disease Case-Control Study Group. JAMA. 1994 Nov 9;272(18):1413-20.

Smith W, Mitchell P, Leeder SR. Dietary fat and fish intake and age-related maculopathy. Arch Ophthalmol. 2000 Mar;118(3):401-4.

Wang, Wei et al. Effect of dietary lutein and zeaxanthin on plasma carotenoids and their transport in lipoproteins in age-related macular degeneration The American Journal of Clinical Nutrition, Volume 85, Issue 3, 762 - 769

Yong JJ, Scott IU, Greenberg PB. Ocular nutritional supplements: are their ingredients and manufacturers' claims evidence-based? Ophthalmology. 2015 Mar;122(3):595-9.

## Multiple Sclerosis

Bjornevik K, Münz C, Cohen JI, Ascherio A. Epstein-Barr virus as a leading cause of multiple sclerosis: mechanisms and implications. Nat Rev Neurol. 2023 Mar;19(3):160-171.

Dobson R, Giovannoni G. Multiple sclerosis-a review. Eur J Neurol. 2019 Jan;26(1):27-40.

Huntley A. et al. Complementary and alternative therapies for treating multiple sclerosis symptoms: a systematic review Complement Ther in Med (2000)

Klineova S, Lublin FD. Clinical Course of Multiple Sclerosis. Cold Spring Harb Perspect Med. 2018 Sep 4;8(9):a028928.

Oh J, Vidal-Jordana A, Montalban X. Multiple sclerosis: clinical aspects. Curr Opin Neurol. 2018 Dec;31(6):752-759.

Riccio P, Rossano R. Nutrition facts in multiple sclerosis. ASN Neuro. 2015 Feb 18;7(1):1759091414568185.

Sintzel MB, Rametta M, Reder AT. Vitamin D and Multiple Sclerosis: A Comprehensive Review. Neurol Ther. 2018 Jun;7(1):59-85.

Stoiloudis P, Kesidou E, Bakirtzis C, et al. The Role of Diet and Interventions on Multiple Sclerosis: A Review. Nutrients. 2022 Mar 9;14(6):1150.

Van der Ploeg, H.M et al. Use of alternative treatments by patients with multiple sclerosis Ned Tijdschr Genesk (1994)

Whitmarsh, Thomas E. Homeopathy in multiple sclerosis Complementary Therapies in Nursing and Midwifery Volume 9, Issue 1, February 2003, Pages 5-9

## Myopia

Biswas S, El Kareh A, Qureshi M, et al. The influence of the environment and lifestyle on myopia. J Physiol Anthropol. 2024 Jan 31;43(1):7.

Carr BJ, Stell WK. Nitric oxide (NO) mediates the inhibition of form-deprivation myopia by atropine in chicks. Sci Rep. 2016;6:9.

Chakraborty R, Ostrin LA, Nickla DL, et al. Circadian rhythms, refractive development, and myopia.Ophthalmic Physiol Opt. 2018;38(3):217-45.

Cooper J, Tkatchenko AV. A review of current concepts of the etiology and treatment of myopia. Eye & Contact Lens. 2018;44:231-47.

Cordain L. Cereal grains: humanity's double-edged sword. World Rev Nutr Diet 1999;84: 19–73.

Coulston AM, Liu GC & Reaven GM. Plasma glucose, insulin and lipid responses to high-carbohydrate low-fat diets in normal humans. Metabolism 1983;32:52–56.

Dreher ML, Davenport AJ. Hass avocado composition and potential health effects. Critical re-views in food science and nutrition. 2013;53:738-50.

Ekdawi NS, Nusz KJ, Diehl NN, et al. The Development of Myopia Among Children with Intermittent Exotropia. American Journal of Ophthalmology. 2010;149(3):503-507.

Flitcroft DI. A model of the contribution of oculomotor and optical factors to emmetropization and myopia. Vision Res. 1998;38(19):2869-79.

Flitcroft D, He M, Jonas J, et al. IMI – Defining and Classifying Myopia: A Proposed Set of Standards for Clinical and Epidemiologic Studies. February 2019.

Fontaine M, Gaucher D, Sauer A, et al. Choroidal thickness and ametropia in children: A longitudinal study. Eur J Ophthalmol 2017;27:730–4.

Fricke TR, Jong M, Naidoo KS et al. Global prevalence of visual impairment associated with myopic macular degeneration and temporal trends from 2000 through 2050: systematic review, me-ta-analysis and modeling. Br J Opththalmol. 2018;102(7):855-62.

Holden BA, Fricke TR, Wilson DA, et al. Global Prevalence of Myopia and High Myopia and Temporal Trends from 2000 through 2050. Ophthalmology. 2016;123(5):1036-1042.

## REFERENCES


Jones LA, Sinnott LT, Mutti DO, et al. Parental history of myopia, sports and outdoor activities, and future myopia. Invest Ophthalmol Vis Sci. 2007;48:3524-32.

Lane BC. Calcium, chromium, protein, sugar and accommodation in myopia. In: Fledelius HC, Alsbirk PH, Goldschmidt E, eds.Documenta Ophthalmologica Proc Series. Vol 28. Third International Conference on Myopia, Copenhagen, The Hague: Dr W Junk Publishers; 1981:141-8.

Lane BC, Aggarwala KR. High myopes are biochemically different from high hyperopes. Myopia 2000: Proceedings of the VIII International Conference on Myopia. 2000;232.

Lane BC. Elevation of intraocular pressure with daily sustained close work stimulus to accommodation: Lowered tissue chromium and dietary deficiency of ascorbic acid (vitamin C). Documenta Ophthalmologica Proceedings Series. Vol. 28; Third International Conference on Myopia, Copenhagen, 1980. H. C. Fledelius, P. H. Alsbirk, and E. Goldschmidt, Eds.The Hague: Dr W Junk Publishers:149-55.

Lingham G, Mackey DA, Lucas R, Yazar S. How does spending time outdoors protect against myopia? A review. Br J Ophthalmol. 2020 May;104(5):593-599.

Liu Y, Wang L, Xu Y, et al. The influence of the choroid on the onset and development of myopia: From perspectives of choroidal thickness and blood flow. Acta Ophthalmol 2021;99:730–8.

McBrien NA, Gentle A. Role of the sclera in the development and pathological complications of myopia. Prog Retin Eye Res 2003;22:307–38.

Min JS, Min BM. The Effect of Alternating Monocular Instillation of 0.125% Atropine in Korean Children with Progressive Myopia. J Clin Med. 2024 Aug 23;13(17):5003.

Morgan IG, Rose KA. Myopia: is the nature-nurture debate finally over? Clin Exp Optom. 2019;102(1):3-17.

Mutti DO, Sinnott LT, Reuter KS, et al. Bifocal lenses in nearsighted kids (BLINK) study group. Peripheral refraction and eye lengths in myopic children in the Bifocal Lenses In Nearsight-ed Kids (BLINK) study. Trans Vis Sci Tech. 2019;8(2):17.

Mutti DO, Hayes JR, Mitchell GL, et al. Refractive error, axial length, and relative peripheral refractive error before and after the onset of myopia. Investigative Ophthalmology and Visual Science. 2007;48(6):2510-2519.

Mutti DO, Jones LA, Moeschberger ML, Zadnik K. AC/A ratio, age, and refractive error in children. Investigative Ophthalmology and Visual Science. 2000;41(9):2469-2478.

Mutti DO, Mitchell GL, Hayes JR, et al. Accommodative lag before and after the onset of myopia. Investigative Ophthalmology and Visual Science. 2006;47(3):837-846.

Mutti DO. Hereditary and environmental contributions to emmetropization and myopia. Optom Vis Sci. 2010 Apr;87(4):255-9.

Ostrin LA, Harb E, Nickla DL, et al. IMI—the dynamic choroid: New insights, challenges, and potential significance for human myopia. *Invest Ophthalmol Vis Sci* 2023;64:4.

Rada JA, Shelton S, Norton TT. The sclera and myopia. Exp Eye Res 2006;82:185–200.

Read SA, Collins MJ, Woodman EC, et al. Axial length changes during accommodation in myopes and emmetropes. *Optom Vis Sci* 2010;87:656–62.

Reiser S, Handler HB, Gardner LB, et al. Isocaloric exchange of dietary starch and sucrose in humans. II. Effect on fasting blood insulin, glucose, and glucagon and on insulin and glucose response to a sucrose load. Am J Clin Nutr 1979;32:2206–16.

Rose KA, Morgan IG, Ip J, et al. Outdoor Activity Reduces the Prevalence of Myopia in Children. Ophthalmology. 2008;115(8):1279-1285.

Rotolo M, Montani G, Martin R. Myopia onset and role of peripheral refraction. Clin Optom (Auckl). 2017;9:105-11.

Rucker FJ, Kruger PB. Cone contributions to signals for accommodation and the relationship to refractive error. Vision Res. 2006;46(19):3079-89.

Rucker FJ, Wallman J. Chicks use changes in illuminance and chromatic contrast as indicators of the sign of defocus. J Vis. 2012;12(6):23, 1-13.

Rucker F, Britton S, Spatcher M, et al. Blue light protects against temporal frequency sensitive refractive changes. Invest Ophthalmol Vis Sci. 2015;56:6121–31.

Saw SM, Chua WH, Gazzard G, et al. Eye growth changes in myopic children in Singapore. Br J Ophthalmol. 2005;89(11):1489-94.

Schaeffel F, Troilo D, Wallman J, et al. Developing eyes that lack accommodation grow to compensate for imposed defocus. Vis Neurosci. 1990;4:177-83.

Smith EL 3rd, Kee CS, Ramamirtham R, et al. Peripheral vision can influence eye growth and refractive development in infant monkeys. Invest Ophthalmol Vis Sci. 2005;46(11):3965-72.

Tideman JWL, Polling JR, Voortman T, et al. Low serum vitamin D is associated with axial length and risk of myopia in young children. Eur J Epidemiol. 2016;31:491-99.

Timucin OB, Arabaci M, Cuce F, et al. The effects of light sources with different spectral structures on ocular axial length in rainbow trout (Oncorhynchus mykiss). Exper Eye Res. 2016;151:212-21.

Torii H, Kurihara T, Seko Y, et al. Violet light exposure can be a preventive strategy against myopia progression. EBioMedicine. 2017; Feb15:210-19.

Wallman J, Winawer J. Homeostasis of eye growth and the question of myopia. Neuron. 2004;43(4):447-68.

Xue CC, Li H, Dong XX, et al Omega-3 Polyunsaturated Fatty Acids as a Protective Factor for Myopia. Am J Ophthalmol. 2024 Dec;268:368-377.

Zadnik K, Sinnott LT, Cotter SA, et al. Prediction of Juvenile-Onset Myopia. JAMA Ophthalmology. 2015;133(6):683-689.

Zhang D, Wang L, Jin L, et al. A review of intraocular pressure (IOP) and axial myopia. *J Ophthalmol* 2022;2022:5626479.

## Nyctalopia

Blankhart DM. Individual intake of food in young children in relation to malnutrition and night blindness. Trop Geogr Med. 1967 Jun;19(2):144-53.

Boyd-Monk H. Vitamin A deficiency and associated eye disease. J Ophthalmic Nurs Technol. 1983 Nov;2(4):159-62.

Mathur GP, Kushwaha KP. Vitamin A deficiency. Indian Pediatr. 1987 Jul;24(7):573-81. PMID: 3500918.

Tiang S, Warne R. Nyctalopia: the sequelae of hypovitaminosis A. BMJ Case Rep. 2010 Aug 26;2010

Verma L, Arora R, Khosla PK, Tiwari HK. Nyctalopia. Indian Pediatr. 1991 May;28(5):575-6.

## Optic Neuritis

Bennett JL. Optic Neuritis. Continuum (Minneap Minn). 2019 Oct;25(5):1236-1264.

Bennett JL, Costello F, Chen JJ, et al. Optic neuritis and autoimmune optic neuropathies: advances in diagnosis and treatment. Lancet Neurol. 2023 Jan;22(1):89-100.

Keyhanian K, Chwalisz BK. The Treatment of Acute Optic Neuritis. Semin Ophthalmol. 2023 Aug;38(6):511-514.

Kraker JA, Chen JJ. An update on optic neuritis. J Neurol. 2023 Oct;270(10):5113-5126.

Plafker SM, Titcomb T, Zyla-Jackson K, Kolakowska A, Wahls T. Overview of diet and autoimmune demyelinating optic neuritis: a narrative review. Immunometabolism (Cobham). 2023 Apr 27;5(2):e00022

Zyla-Jackson K, Walton DA, Plafker KS, et al. Dietary protection against the visual and motor deficits induced by experimental autoimmune encephalomyelitis. Front Neurol. 2023 Mar 2;14:1113954.

## Pinguecula

Bell A. Pinguecula. J Vis Commun Med. 2006 Jun;29(2):82-3.

Mudhar HS. Update on conjunctival pathology. Indian J Ophthalmol. 2017 Sep;65(9):797-807.

Perkins E. S. The association between pinguecula, sunlight and cataract. Ophthalmic Research. 1985;17(6):325–330.

Somnath A, Tripathy K. Pinguecula. 2023 Aug 25. In: StatPearls [Internet]. Treasure Island (FL): StatPearls Publishing; 2025 Jan

## Pterygium

Celeva Markovska V, Stankovic Babic G, Zdravkovska Jankuloska M. Comparative study of pterygium surgery. Prilozi. 2011;32(2):273-87.

Chu WK, Choi HL, Bhat AK, Jhanji V. Pterygium: new insights. Eye (Lond). 2020 Jun;34(6):1047-1050.

Hacıoğlu D, Erdöl H. Developments and current approaches in the treatment of pterygium. Int Ophthalmol. 2017 Aug;37(4):1073-1081.

He S, Wu Z. Biomarkers in the Occurrence and Development of Pterygium. Ophthalmic Res. 2022;65(5):481-492.

Kaufman SC, Jacobs DS, Lee WB, et al. Options and adjuvants in surgery for pterygium: a report by the American Academy of Ophthalmology. Ophthalmology. 2013 Jan;120(1):201-8.

## Retinitis Pigmentosa

Bonilla L, Espina M, Severino P, Cano A, Ettcheto M, Camins A, García ML, Souto EB, Sánchez-López E. Lipid Nanoparticles for the Posterior Eye Segment. Pharmaceutics. 2021 Dec 31;14(1):90

Jing H, Nie M, Wang X, et al. Lutein combined with EGCG improved retinitis pigmentosa against *N*-methyl-*N* nitrosourea-induced. Food Funct. 2023 Oct 30;14(21):9554-9566.

Liu W, Liu S, Li P, Yao K. Retinitis Pigmentosa: Progress in Molecular Pathology and Biotherapeutical Strategies. Int J Mol Sci. 2022 Apr 28;23(9):4883.

Fahim A. Retinitis pigmentosa: recent advances and future directions in diagnosis and management. Curr Opin Pediatr. 2018 Dec;30(6):725-733.

Gonçalves PB, Sodero ACR, Cordeiro Y. Green Tea Epigallocatechin-3-gallate (EGCG) Targeting Protein Misfolding in Drug Discovery for Neurodegenerative Diseases. Biomolecules. 2021 May 20;11(5):767.

He Y, Zhang Y, Su G. Recent advances in treatment of retinitis pigmentosa. Curr Stem Cell Res Ther. 2015;10(3):258-65.

Maher P. The potential of flavonoids for the treatment of neurodegenerative diseases. Int. J. Mol. Sci. 2019;20 doi: 10.3390/ijms20123056.

Payne A, Nahashon S, Taka E, et al. Epigallocatechin-3-Gallate (EGCG): New Therapeutic Perspectives for Neuroprotection, Aging, and Neuroinflammation for the Modern Age. Biomolecules. 2022 Feb 25;12(3):371.

Ramdas WD, Schouten JSAG, Webers CAB. The Effect of Vitamins on Glaucoma: A Systematic Review and Meta-Analysis. Nutrients. 2018 Mar 16;10(3):359

Vingolo EM, Mascolo S, Miccichè F, Manco G. Retinitis Pigmentosa: From Pathomolecular Mechanisms to Therapeutic Strategies. Medicina (Kaunas). 2024 Jan 22;60(1):189.

Zhao L, Hou C, Yan N. Neuroinflammation in retinitis pigmentosa: Therapies targeting the innate immune system. Front Immunol. 2022 Oct 27;13:1059947.

# Part III: Nutritional Approaches

## Diets

Agrón E, Mares J, Chew EY, Keenan TDL; AREDS2 Research Group. Adherence to a Mediterranean Diet and Geographic Atrophy Enlargement Rate: Age-Related Eye Disease Study 2 Report 29. Ophthalmol Retina. 2022 Sep;6(9):762-770.

Barrea L, Muscogiuri G, Frias-Toral E, et al. A. Nutrition and immune system: from the Mediterranean diet to dietary supplementary through the microbiota. Crit Rev Food Sci Nutr. 2021;61(18):3066-3090.

## REFERENCES


Bastard JP, et al. Recent advances in the relationship between obesity, inflammation, and insulin resistance. Eur Cytokine Netw. 2006 Mar;17(1):4-12

Cordain, Loren (Author) The Paleo Diet Revised: Lose Weight and Get Healthy by Eating the Foods You Were Designed to Eat – December 7, 2010

Challa HJ, Bandlamudi M, Uppaluri KR. Paleolithic Diet. [Updated 2023 Jul 4]. In: StatPearls [Internet]. Treasure Island (FL): StatPearls Publishing; 2025 Jan-. Available from: https://www.ncbi.nlm.nih.gov/books/NBK482457/

Danescu LG, Levy S, Levy J. Vitamin D and diabetes mellitus. Endocrine. 2009 Feb;24(1):11-7

De Lorgeril MD, et al. Mediterranean diet, traditional risk factors, and the rate of cardiovascular complications after myocardial infarction: Final report of the Lyon diet heart study. Circulation, 99(6): (1999);779–785.

Du X, Edelstain D, Brownlee M. Oral benfotiamine plus alpha-lipoic acid normalizes complication-causing pathways in type 1 diabetes. Diabetologia. 2008 Oct;51(10):1930-2

Economic Costs of Diabetes in the U.S. in 2022 Diabetes Care, Vol. 47, No. 1, January 2024

Esposito K, Giugliano D. The metabolic syndrome and inflammation:association or causation? Nutr Metab Cardiovasc Dis. 2004 Oct;14(5):228–32.

Kahn HA, Hiller R. Blindness caused by diabetic retinopathy. Am J Ophthalmol. 1974 Jul;78(1):58-67.

Kiani AK, Medori MC, Bonetti G, et al. Modern vision of the Mediterranean diet. J Prev Med Hyg. 2022 Oct 17;63(2 Suppl 3):E36-E43.

Molina-Leyva I, Molina-Leyva A, Riquelme-Gallego B, et al. Effectiveness of Mediterranean Diet Implementation in Dry Eye Parameters: A Study of PREDIMED-PLUS Trial. Nutrients. 2020 May 1;12(5):1289.

Nutrition Recommendations and Interventions for Diabetes: A position statement of the American Diabetes Association Diabetes Care January 2008 vol. 31 no. Supplement 1 S61-S78

Robinson LE, Buchholz AC, Mazurak VC. Inflammation, obesity, and fatty acid metabolism: influence of n-3 polyunsaturated fatty acids on factors contributing to metabolic syndrome. Appl Physiol Nutr Metab. 2007 Dec;32)6):1008-24

Román GC, Jackson RE, Gadhia R, et al. Mediterranean diet: The role of long-chain ω-3 fatty acids in fish; polyphenols in fruits, vegetables, cereals, coffee, tea, cacao and wine; probiotics and vitamins in prevention of stroke, age-related cognitive decline, and Alzheimer disease. Rev Neurol (Paris). 2019 Dec;175(10):724-741

Sbai O, Torrisi F, Fabrizio FP, et al. Effect of the Mediterranean Diet (MeDi) on the Progression of Retinal Disease: A Narrative Review. Nutrients. 2024 Sep 19;16(18):3169.

Volek, J; Yancy, WS, Jr; Gower, B; et al. Expert consensus on nutrition and lower-carbohydrate diets: An evidence- and equity-based approach to dietary guidance Front. Nutr. , 28 February 2024 Sec. Nutrition and Metabolism Volume 11 - 2024

Wu Y, Xie Y, Yuan Y, et al. The Mediterranean Diet and Age-Related Eye Diseases: A Systematic Review. Nutrients. 2023 Apr 23;15(9):2043.

Zhu Q, Liu X, Qu Y, et al. Neuroprotective effects of healthful plant-based diets on retinal structure: insights from a large cohort. J Nutr Health Aging. 2025 Jan;29(1):100431

Zohoori FV. Chapter 1: Nutrition and Diet. Monogr Oral Sci. 2020;28:1-13.

## Nutrition for the Diabetic Patient

Goday A, Bellido D, Sajoux I, et al. Short-term safety, tolerability and efficacy of a very low-calorie-ketogenic diet interventional weight loss program versus hypocaloric diet in patients with type 2 diabetes mellitus. Nutr Diabetes. 2016 Sep 19;6(9):e230.

Hannon BA, Fairfield WD, Adams B, et al. Use and abuse of dietary supplements in persons with diabetes. Nutr Diabetes. 2020 Apr 27;10(1):14.

Henry CJ, Kaur B, Quek RYC. Chrononutrition in the management of diabetes. Nutr Diabetes. 2020 Feb 19;10(1):6.

Li C, Zhang Y, Wang Y, et al. Imaging-based body fat distribution and diabetic retinopathy in general US population with diabetes: an NHANES analysis (2003-2006 and 2011-2018). Nutr Diabetes. 2024 Jul 14;14(1):53.

Podadera-Herreros A, Arenas-de Larriva AP, Gutierrez-Mariscal FM, et al. Mediterranean diet as a strategy for preserving kidney function in patients with coronary heart disease with type 2 diabetes and obesity: a secondary analysis of CORDIOPREV randomized controlled trial. Nutr Diabetes. 2024 May 16;14(1):27.

Shih KC, Lam KS, Tong L. A systematic review on the impact of diabetes mellitus on the ocular surface. Nutr Diabetes. 2017 Mar 20;7(3):e251.

Yuan X, Wang J, Yang S, et al. Effect of the ketogenic diet on glycemic control, insulin resistance, and lipid metabolism in patients with T2DM: a systematic review and meta-analysis. Nutr Diabetes. 2020 Nov 30;10(1):38.

## Eye-Gut Connection

Ciurariu E, Tirziu AT, Varga NI, Hirtie B, Alexandru A, Ivan CS, Nicolescu L. Short-Chain Fatty Acids and the Gut-Retina Connection: A Systematic Review. Int J Mol Sci. 2025 Mar 10;26(6):2470.

Huang L, Hong Y, Fu X, Tan H, Chen Y, Wang Y, Chen D. The role of the microbiota in glaucoma. Mol Aspects Med. 2023 Dec;94:101221.

Jin Q, Wang S, Yao Y, et al. The gut-eye axis: from brain neurodegenerative diseases to age-related macular degeneration. Neural Regen Res. 2025 Oct 1;20(10):2741-2757.

Mi Y, Chen K, Lin S, et al. Lactobacillaceae-mediated eye-brain-gut axis regulates high myopia-related anxiety: from the perspective of predictive, preventive, and personalized medicine. EPMA J. 2024 Nov 26;15(4):573-585

Rowan S, Taylor A. The Role of Microbiota in Retinal Disease. Adv Exp Med Biol. 2018;1074:429-435.

Scholz R, Langmann T. Gut flora connects obesity with pathological angiogenesis in the eye. EMBO Mol Med. 2016 Dec 1;8(12):1361-1363.

Shivaji S. Connect between gut microbiome and diseases of the human eye. J Biosci. 2019 Oct;44(5):110.

Zhao Y, Qiu P, Shen T. Gut microbiota and eye diseases: A review. Medicine (Baltimore). 2024 Sep 27;103(39):e39866.

## Herbal Therapy

Ahmadi A. The Beneficial Roles of Herbal Medicine and Natural Product in CNS Disorders and Neurodegeneration. Curr Pharm Des. 2021;27(3):331.

Fraunfelder FW. Ocular side effects from herbal medicines and nutritional supplements. Am J Ophthalmol. 2004 Oct;138(4):639-47.

Gossman CA, Christie J, Webster MK, et al. Neuroprotective Strategies in Glaucoma. Curr Pharm Des. 2016;22(14):2178-92.

Kumar V. Potential medicinal plants for CNS disorders: an overview. Phytother Res. 2006 Dec;20(12):1023-35.

Pang GM, Li FX, Yan Y, et al. Herbal medicine in the treatment of patients with type 2 diabetes mellitus. Chin Med J (Engl). 2019 Jan 5;132(1):78-85.

Vitiello L, Capasso L, Cembalo G, et al. Herbal and Natural Treatments for the Management of the Glaucoma: An Update. Biomed Res Int. 2023 Nov 17;2023:3105251.

West AL, Oren GA, Moroi SE. Evidence for the use of nutritional supplements and herbal medicines in common eye diseases. Am J Ophthalmol. 2006 Jan;141(1):157-66

Wilkinson JT, Fraunfelder FW. Use of herbal medicines and nutritional supplements in ocular disorders: an evidence-based review. Drugs. 2011 Dec 24;71(18):2421-34.

## Homeopathy

Moffat JL. Homeopathic Therapeutics in Ophthalmology. Jain Publishers, New Delhi, 1982

Murphy R. Homeopathic Medical repertory: A Modern Alphabetic repertory (Hahnemann Academy of North America, 1993

## Ocular Side Effects of Systemic Medications

Armaly M.F., Becker B. Intraocular pressure response to topical corticosteroids. Fed. Proc. 1965;24:1274–1278

Cai S., Liu T.Y.A., Arevalo J.F. Evolution of Ellipsoid Zone Abnormalities on Optical Coherence Tomography Associated With Niacin Maculopathy. JAMA Ophthalmol. 2019;137:849–851.

Green MB, Duker JS. Adverse Ocular Effects of Systemic Medications. Life (Basel). 2023 Feb 28;13(3):660.

Mandal P., Gupta A., Fusi-Rubiano W., A Keane P., Yang Y. Fingolimod: Therapeutic mechanisms and ocular adverse effects. Eye. 2016;31:232–240.

Wang M.Y., Sadun A.A. Drug-Related Mitochondrial Optic Neuropathies. J. Neuro-Ophthalmol. 2013;33:172–178.

Wu A., Khawaja A.P., Pasquale L.R., Stein J.D. A review of systemic medications that may modulate the risk of glaucoma. Eye. 2019;34:12–28.

## Drug-Nutrient Interactions

Chan LN. Drug-nutrient interaction in clinical nutrition. Curr Opin Clin Nutr Metab Care. 2002 May;5(3):327-32.

Chan LN. Drug-nutrient interactions. JPEN J Parenter Enteral Nutr. 2013 Jul;37(4):450-9.

England E, Cheng C. Nutrition: Micronutrients. FP Essent. 2024 Apr;539:13-17.

Felípez L, Sentongo TA. Drug-induced nutrient deficiencies. Pediatr Clin North Am. 2009 Oct;56(5):1211-24.

Genser D. Food and drug interaction: consequences for the nutrition/health status. Ann Nutr Metab. 2008;52 Suppl 1:29-32.

Harvie M. Nutritional supplements and cancer: potential benefits and proven harms. Am Soc Clin Oncol Educ Book. 2014:e478-86.

Thomas JA. Drug-nutrient interactions. Nutr Rev. 1995 Oct;53(10):271-82.

Trovato A, Nuhlicek DN, Midtling JE. Drug-nutrient interactions. Am Fam Physician. 1991 Nov;44(5):1651-8.

# ABOUT THE AUTHOR

**Jeffrey R. Anshel**, OD, received his Bachelor of Science degree in visual science and his Doctorate of Optometry from the Illinois College of Optometry. After his service in the US Navy, Dr. Anshel went into private practice, offering his patients nutrition and alternative therapies as part of their vision care. Dr. Anshel is the creator of the "20-20-20" rule for computer display users. He lectures internationally and has written eight books on eye care, including Smart Medicine for Your Eyes and What You Must Know About Age-Related Macular Degeneration. Dr. Anshel is a Fellow of the American Academy of Optometry and currently maintains a consulting practice in Kauai, Hawaii.

www.ingramcontent.com/pod-product-compliance
Lightning Source LLC
LaVergne TN
LVHW080023210926
848481LV00011B/3096
* 9 7 8 0 7 5 7 0 0 5 4 5 9 *